Advance Praise for Sgt. Rory Miller's *Meditations on Violence:*

Simply put *Meditations on Violence* tells the truth. Sgt. Rory Miller will wipe away any fantasy you have about fighting. Fighting and violence will tolerate no lies—especially the ones you tell yourself. The more you read the more you will realize that the stupid, "Monkey Dance" you do is meaningless. The words, the displays, they are all predictable, and Sgt. Miller has your number.

–**Kris Wilder**, martial artist, author

Kris holds black belt-level ranks in three arts: Tae Kwon Do (2nd Degree), Kodokan Judo (1st Degree) and Goju-Ryu Karate (4th Degree), instructor West Seattle Karate Academy

Author:

- *The Way of Sanchin Kata*

Co-Author:

- *The Little Black Book of Violence*

Miller uses his words like a samurai sword, cutting through flesh, bone, and sinew, directly into the heart of the matter—your ego and life-long distorted illusions about yourself, violence, and ways in which you prepare yourself for today's battlefield—the street, where illusion and reality clash. Will you be a victim of your own training flaws? This book is a wake-up call to all those practicing, and especially those teaching, martial arts who think that "self-defense" training in the dojo actually constitutes proper preparation for real life encounters on the street. Miller says: "A real fight for your life is NOTHING like sparring." Indeed it isn't.

–**Sgt. Alan D. Arsenault**, 27-year veteran
Vancouver P.D., martial artist, author

Alan is the Executive Director of the famed Odd Squad www.oddsquad.com

Author:

- Chin Na in Ground Fighting

This book is a refreshingly frank, honest, and in-depth assessment of violence. As a corrections officer, Miller tangles with hard-core predators for a living. He routinely survives brutal encounters that would leave the average person physically shattered and emotionally wrecked. Miller's insights on how to make self-defense work and overcome subconscious resistance to meeting violence with violence could very well save your life one day. Learn how to think critically about the subject, determine how to evaluate sources of knowledge, and understand how to identify strategies and select tactics to deal with violence effectively. This extraordinarily well-written book is packed with interesting, informative, and, most importantly, useful information.

–**Lawrence A. Kane,** martial artist,
author, security supervisor

Lawrence is responsible for fan safety during college and professional football games at a Pac-10 stadium.

Author:

- *Surviving Armed Assaults*
- *Martial Arts Instruction*

Co-Author:

- *The Little Black Book of Violence*
- *The Way to Black Belt*
- *The Way of Kata*

A must read book for LEO's (Law Enforcement Officer's), martial artists, and anyone interesting in learning about the complexities of violence. Not only do I highly recommend this book, but will be required reading for my students a well.

–**Antonio B. Urena,** Detective Sergeant,
martial artist

Antonio holds 7th Degree black belt in Okinawan Karate, is a NJ certified defensive tactics, firearms, assault rifle, and subgun instructor, a SWAT team squad leader and police sniper.

This is the finest self-defense book it has ever been my pleasure to read, and I have read quite a few. I feel it is a seminal work, and that is not praise I bandy about lightly. In fact, I hope that my many friends in the self-defense publishing world forgive me for putting Mr. Miller's book above theirs in my particular pecking order. It is simply that good.

This book is not a book that will teach you Angry Monkey Kung Fu or the Tiger Claws An Ox technique. In fact, the book is very short on technique offered, which is its true strength. There are innumerable books out there that are technique driven. That's not the problem. What is lacking, and most sorely needed, is exploration on the realities of human-on-human violence. What drives it, how do you survive it, and how and what can we learn from it.

As a LEO I've been in many, many use of force incidents, a couple of shootings, and had more incidents that had the potential to become violent but didn't. In very few of them did any particular technique come to me to "Save The Day." What served me much better was the understanding of what was happening, recognizing it as it happened, and not letting the fear and adrenaline keep me from acting, even if the acting in question was simply talking the situation down.

Hopefully your particular art has given you the physical tools needed to affect your self-defense. Technique is important, no doubt, but any defense scenario is much more than a series of techniques thrown in a vacuum. This book will fill in those gaps—all the other stuff that goes along with it. And that is truly where the art of self-defense lies, outside of technique.

–**M. Guthrie**, Federal Air Marshal

Guthrie is a fifteen-year veteran of LEO (Law Enforcement Officer) work, including local LEO (gang unit), and U.S. Border Patrol.

In the world of Martial Arts, there are many books written by experts in their various arts. While these authors are experts in their own martial disciple, very few can make the claim that they are experts in combat in the real world. Yes, contrary to popular belief, just because you are an expert in the martial arts does not make you an expert in self-defense or real world combat. However, everyone once in a while along comes someone who is both an expert in martial arts, and in the area of real world combat. Even more rare, is the person who has taken their years of training in the martial arts and adapted it to the realities of a violent world. Rory Miller, an experienced martial artist and corrections officer is such a person.

In his book, *Meditations on Violence—A Comparison of Martial Arts Training & Real World Violence*, he explores the reality of violence and how to survive it. Exposing the myths that surround violence and combat, Rory gives the reader a stark look into the real world, one that he must confront every day when he goes to work. Rather than a "how to" book filled with lots of cool pictures, his book informs the reader of the psychology, mindset, and strategies that will keep you alive, and suggests methods that will better prepare you for the real world. I highly recommend this book for anyone who may have to confront the reality of violence, especially martial artists who are often in the most need of a reality check.

–**Robert Carver**, martial artist, President US Martial Arts Federation, Founder of BudoSeek! Martial Arts Community (www.budoseek.net), member of the Board of Directors for the U.S. Ju-Jitsu Federation

Robert is a former U.S. Marine, 35 years of martial arts experience, 6th Dan – Heiwashin Kai Jujutsu, 6th Dan – U.S. Jujitsu (USJJF National System), 5th Dan – Seki Ryu Jujitsu, 5th Dan – Judo, 3rd Dan – Shorinryu Karate, 2nd Dan – Minami Ryu Jujutsu, Certified Master Instructor, United States Ju-Jitsu Federation.

One of the best books on self-protection ever written! This book is packed with vital information and is certain to be of great benefit to all martial artists wise enough to read it. Outstanding!

–**Iain Abernethy**, British Combat Association
Senior Coach, martial artist, author
www.iainabernethy.com

Iain holds 5th Dan Waydo Ryu Karate, is a member of Combat Hall of Fame, and a former U.K. national level kata judge.

Author:

- *Bunkai Jutsu*
- *Mental Strength*

A fresh voice writing from the trenches on the realities of real fighting. Listen to him. [This book] sheds insight on the psychology and physicality of dealing with people who want to rip your head off. [If you are really serious about self-defense, you'll want to] learn from a veteran corrections officer the ugly reality of real fighting as opposed to how it's taught in too many strip mall dojos.

Every martial artist, every cop and every corrections officer should read this book.

–**Loren Christensen**, (ret) police officer,
Portland P.D., martial artist, author

Loren is a 7th Dan black belt, Vietnam veteran and author of 35 books. www.lwcbooks.com. Loren was named by Black Belt *magazine as "one of the top twenty toughest Men on Planet Earth."*

Author:

- *Solo Training*
- *Fighters Fact Book*
- *On Combat* (co-author with Lt. Col. Dave Grossman)

The **difference between theory and practice** is in theory there is no difference. Unfortunately, countless law enforcement and correctional officers, security professionals and private citizens have discovered this also applies to the training they have received in the safety of a martial arts school (or academy) and the realities of applying that training in a live-fire situation.

The reason this transition is so difficult is because surviving physical violence is so much more than just punching, kicking, or pulling a trigger. From the safety of training, these elements seem like small obstacles that will be easily overcome. Unfortunately, in a live-fire situation those small obstacles can become huge canyons. Rory Miller's book is not only a fantastic introduction to what you will face in a violent situation, but it provides keen insights and concepts that even an experienced operative will find useful in staying safe in a dangerous occupation

–**Marc 'Animal' MacYoung,** martial artist, self-defense consultant www.nononsenseselfdefense.com, author

Author:
- *A Professional's Guide to Ending Violence Quickly*
- *Cheap Shots, Ambushes and Other Lessons*

MEDITATIONS
ON VIOLENCE

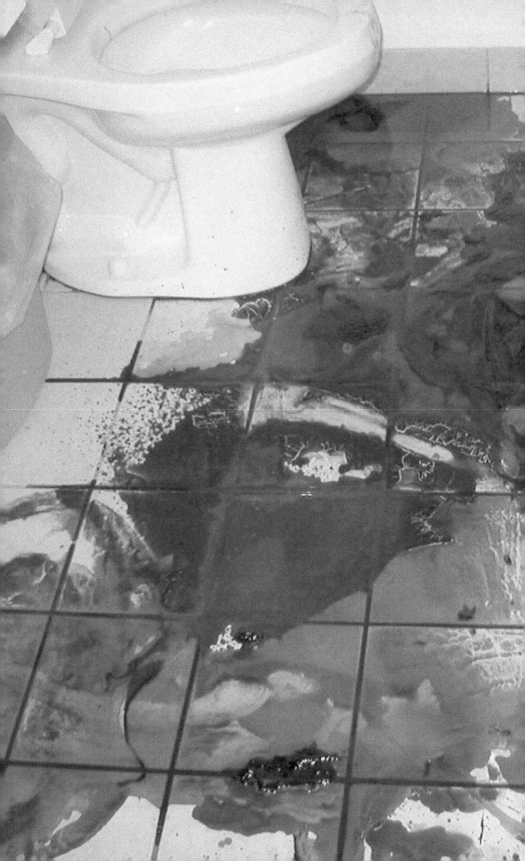

MEDITATIONS ON VIOLENCE

A Comparison of
Martial Arts Training &
Real World Violence

Sergeant Rory Miller

YMAA Publication Center
Boston, Mass. USA

YMAA Publication Center, Inc.
Main Office
  PO Box 480
  Wolfeboro, NH 03894
  1-800-669-8892 • www.ymaa.com • info@ymaa.com

Cover Design: Richard Rossiter
Editing: Tim Comrie

Photo on previous page courtesy of Critical Care BioRecovery, LLC

ISBN-13: 978-1-59439-118-7

ISBN-10: 1-59439-118-1

Printed in USA.

20191213

Publisher's Cataloging in Publication

Miller, Rory, 1964-
    Meditations on violence : a comparison of martial arts training & real
    world violence / Rory Miller. -- 1st ed. -- Boston, Mass. : YMAA
    Publication Center, c2008.

        p. ; cm.
        ISBN: 978-1-59439-118-7
        Includes bibliographical references and index.

        1. Martial arts--Psychological aspects. 2. Violence--
    Psychological aspects. 3. Fighting (Psychology) I. Title.

    GV1102.P75 M55 2008   2008927616
    796.8/092--dc22   0806

Warning: Readers are encouraged to be aware of all appropriate local and national laws relating to self-defense, reasonable force, and the use of weaponry, and act in accordance with all applicable laws at all times. Neither the authors nor the publisher assume any responsibility for the use or misuse of information contained in this book.

Nothing in this document constitutes a legal opinion nor should any of its contents be treated as such. While the authors believe that everything herein is accurate, any questions regarding specific self-defense situations, legal liability, and/or interpretation of federal, state, or local laws should always be addressed by an attorney at law.

When it comes to martial arts, self-defense, and related topics, no text, no matter how well written, can substitute for professional, hands-on instruction. These materials should be used *for academic study only.*

CONTENTS

FOREWORD

By Steven Barnes

There is a "gap" between reality and fantasy, and that "gap" is where the novelist plays. Whether the reality of day to day life in marriage as opposed to the fantasy world of "falling in love," the reality of the workaday world as opposed to the fantasy of "making it big," or the reality of life and death combat as opposed to the fantasies of battlefield glory.

The gaps between these things are the meat of my profession. Because so few of us actually place our lives in jeopardy, ever face the reality of combat, or self-defense, of facing an aggressive human being, or discovering our own potential for violence, we are endlessly fascinated by images of the men and women who can and have done such things. We make them into heroes, we study them in books, we are hypnotized by their images on thirty-foot high movie screens, and pay those who can convincingly portray them staggering sums of money.

And behind much of our fascination is a question: what would I be in that context? Could I cope? And what would I become if I did? What would happen if I could not?

One of those who portrayed this hyper-effective fighting machine stereotype was, of course, Bruce Lee, and after *Enter the Dragon*, legions of young men swamped martial arts schools all over the world, seeking to be strong, to be brave, to be capable—to, in other words, deal with their fear that they would not be *able*. Or to feed their hunger to learn what that mysterious creature lurking in the back of their subconscious was really all about.

I remember during the early 1980's, when training at the Filipino Kali Academy, a school maintained by Danny Inosanto and Richard Bustillo (two former Lee students), that every time a new class opened up, we'd be flooded by the LBKs—Little Blond Kids. They came in the doors with their eyes filled with dreams of martial glory. And we knew that the instant it got real, the instant we put on the gloves and actually started whacking each other, 90% of them would flee.

And friends, sparring in the school has a very limited application to what happens on the streets. Those of us who wanted to learn how to apply what we learned in an academic context to a real life and death situation studied texts by ancient samurai, killer monks, warriors of every culture—those who had actually been and done. We struggled to grasp the difference between fantasy and reality, between theory and application. Because the gap between them could cost us our lives.

Could we do it? And what if we could not?

I met Rory Miller about fifteen years ago, and was immediately impressed by an odd fluidity of movement that told me that he had endured long and intense practice in some effective physical discipline. I suspected martial applications. Over time, I learned about his background, and that his profession as a Corrections Officer placed him in the peculiar position of, as he said at the time, having "A fight a day."

Every day? Against some of the most dangerous and desperate members of our society? This was not a theoretician. But more than his obvious skill, what impressed me was the quality of his relationship with his lady, Kami. Their clear and obvious love told me that he had been able to find a way to engage in violence at a level most martial artists, most people, cannot even dream—without losing his soul.

Because he is both classically trained *and* the survivor of literally countless all-out confrontations, Rory has the absolute right and responsibility to share his impressions of the difference between theory and application. What works and what will get you killed. What attitudes and illusions are harbored by those of us who don't have to face the animals who ENJOY hurting, killing, raping, maiming. What is that space? Where do you have to go inside yourself to survive?

I believe that his training, environment, and inclination created a "Perfect Storm" of martial awareness, in which he has attained a kind of clarity about these things that is a hallmark of those on the road to enlightenment. Very few human beings would be willing to pay the price he has paid, or be capable of paying it even if they were willing.

That he is willing to report back what he has learned is an act of love and social responsibility. I have the very highest respect for Rory and what he has to say about the "gap" between martial arts as taught and conceptualized, and survival in the crucible of actual combat. In other words, how he stepped through the fire without being utterly destroyed by the flame.

Meditations on Violence—A Comparison of Martial Arts Training & Real World Violence is not a joke, or a fantasy, or a screed written to salve the ego of some wannabe. I've met the men who work with Rory, and they are tough, hard, guys—and they adore him. They know that what he knows, and who he is, has kept them alive to return to their lives and families.

You hold in your hands a document long in incubation, the musings of a modern warrior on a topic central to mankind's survival since the first dawn.

Can I? And if I can, how? And who will I be? What MUST I be, to protect my life, my values, my family?

There are few questions more important than these.

Here, in these pages, are the results of one man's quest for answers.

It's the real thing.

Steven Barnes
Southern California
August 1, 2007

Steven Barnes is a N.Y. Times bestselling novelist and former Kung-Fu columnist for Black Belt *magazine.*

ACKNOWLEDGMENTS

This is a book about many things and I was helped by many people from many different worlds. Cops and criminals, friends, trainers, authors, and students have all helped with this work—some directly with the manuscript and very, very many with opening my eyes to different parts of the world.

From the world of martial arts: Sensei Mike Moore and Sensei Wolfgang Dill set my foundation. Sensei Dave Sumner introduced me to *Sosuishi-ryu*, which became my core. Whatever I am as a fighter, Dave created. And Paul McRedmond (Mac)—has carried the torch from there, showing me new depths and urging me toward a purer intention. I can never thank you enough.

From the world of crime and cops, there are too many names. The guys who wore the cuffs taught me as much as the ones who put them on. To the bad guys—thanks for the lessons, now go forth and sin no more. By name—Sgt. Bill Gatzke taught me what it was to be a sergeant; Phil Anderchuk taught me how to plan. C.D. Bishop trusted my judgment. Lt. Inman made me do the parts of the job I hated. Deputy U.S. Marshal J. Jones taught a new level of precision. Thank you all. And most of all, to all CERT members past and present—you've always had my back and demanded my best. NPNBW!

Living is one thing, writing it down is something else. Mary Rosenblum taught me that writing well was a skill. With the help of Mike Moscoe Shepherd she had a big hand in turning a barely literate jail guard into something of a writer. I thank them both, but maybe the readers are the ones who should be grateful.

Every new book gets read many times by many people before it ever sees print—so for encouragement, finding the big holes and helping translate things from my special private language into basic human words: Dana Sheets, Riku Ylonen, Jeff Burger, Jim Raistrick, Mark Jones, and Lawrence Kane. Special thanks to Kris Wilder—without your impetuosity, bad timing, and total disregard for my comfort level, this might never have been seen by a publisher. Thanks, pal.

A few cross over—Roz, Sonia Orin Lyris, and Drew learned and taught both and went over the drafts as well.

Thanks to David Ripianzi and Tim Comrie for making this whole manuscript-to-book process so easy. Easy for me, anyway. Making it look easy takes a true professional.

The last part is personal. Through everything, Kami has the immense responsibility of keeping me sane and holding me to my promise to always be one of the good guys. Thanks. No matter how bad it gets, I've always been able to look at you and know that on balance the world is a good place.

Lastly, to Norma Joyce Miller. The first steps are the most important. As I promised as a wee child, this first book is for you.

INTRODUCTION: METAPHORS

People are weird. They have an almost infinite ability to learn and communicate. At the same time, this amazing ability is used as much for fantasy and entertainment as it is for information and survival. Take, for example, the rhinoceros and the unicorn.

The rhinoceros is a real beast, an animal native to Asia and Africa. It is large, formidable, and familiar to most of us from pictures or visits to the zoo. What do we really know about rhinoceros? Are they grazers or browsers? Do they live in big herds, family groups, or roam the savannah alone? In the movie *The Gods Must be Crazy,* we learned that the rhinoceros doesn't like fire and will stamp out a campfire. Is that true? I have no idea. Look at how little we know, and how little we know with confidence, about this beast that really exists and is truly dangerous.

The unicorn derived from the rhinoceros. Over time and distance and by word of mouth, the reality of the rhinoceros slowly changed into the myth of the unicorn. This process has been so powerful that everyone knows many, many facts about the unicorn. It has the beard of a goat, cloven hooves, and a single horn. It kills elephants by impaling and is strong enough to hurl the elephant over its head, yet it can be tamed and captured by a virgin. We know all these "facts" about the unicorn, but there is only one true fact to know:

The unicorn is imaginary.

Unicorns are mythical, yet we know so much about them. The rhinoceros is real and, except for a few experts, we know so little.

There is a parallel between the unicorn and violence. Just as travelers' tales passing from person to person and place to place and century to century managed to morph the reality of the rhinoceros into the fable of the unicorn, the insular tradition and history of each *dojo* has morphed a primal understanding of violence into the modern ritual of martial arts. Just as the grey and wrinkled skin of the rhinoceros has become the glossy white coat of the unicorn, the smells, and sounds, and gut-wrenching fear of close-up personal violence has somehow spawned the beautiful cinema of the action adventure movie and the crisp precision of the martial arts.

In today's world, who are the real experts on violence?

The Priests of Mars. The minute you don a black belt, the minute you step in front of a class to teach, you are seen as an expert on violence. It doesn't matter if you have absorbed a complete philosophical system with your martial art. It doesn't matter if the art gave you, for the first time, the confidence to view the world as a pacifist. It doesn't matter if you studied as a window to another age and culture. It doesn't matter that you have found enlightenment in *kata* or learned to blend in harmony with the force of your attacker. It doesn't matter because you are about to teach a martial art, an art dedicated to Mars, the God of War. A MARtial art. Even if somewhere over the years you have lost sight of this, your students have not. You wear a black belt. You are an expert on violence. You kick ass. You are a priest of Mars.

The simple truth is that many of these experts, these priests of Mars, have no experience with violence. Very, very few have experienced enough to critically look at what they have been taught, and what they are teaching, and separate the myth from the reality.

The Super Star. Do you ever notice that weight lifters don't look like boxers? For that matter, if you watch fencing matches you see a lot of tall skinny guys, Judo matches tend to be won by short, stocky *judoka*—basically, none of them look like body builders. But action stars usually do. Unless they want to appeal to the goth/techno market, in which case they are really skinny, pale-complected, and wear a lot of black.

The idea is the same—pretty sells. In the media world, everything is about attraction. The fighters look pretty, not the gnarled, scarred up, sometimes toothless fighters that I know. The fights look pretty, too— you can actually see the action and even identify specific techniques.

They are paced for dramatic content. A movie fight doesn't end when the hero or villain would naturally be lying in a pool of bloody vomit, clutching his abdomen and gurgling. It ends at the moment the director thinks the audience is hyped and not bored yet.

Even when they try to be realistic, it's about the spectacle. The very fact that the camera can see what is going on is unrealistic. In smoke and dust and rain and the melee of bodies or the flash of gunfire, the person right in the middle of it can't reliably tell what is going on.

And the fighting caters to the audience's idea of fair. It's almost always a close fight to the very end, won by a slim margin...I'll tell you right now that as a public servant who runs a tactical team if I ever, ever play it fair, if I ever take chances with my men or hostages in order to cater to some half-assed idea of fair play, fire me. Fair doesn't happen in real life, not if the bad guys have anything to say about it and not if the professional good guys do, either. I always wanted to see a movie with Conan talking shit in a bar and looking down to see a knife sticking out of his stomach with no idea how it got there.

The Story. Maybe this is a metaphor, maybe it is a model: Things are what they are. Violence is what it is. You are you, no more and no less—but humans can't leave simple things alone.

One of the ways we complicate things is by telling stories, especially stories about ourselves. This story we tell ourselves is our identity. The essence of every good story is conflict. So our identity, the central character of this story that we tell ourselves, is based largely on how we deal with conflict. If there has been little conflict in the life, the character, our identity, is mostly fictional.

I present this as a warning. You are what you are, not what you think you are. Violence is what it is, not necessarily what you have been told.

This book is about violence, especially about the difference between violence as it exists "in the wild" and violence as it is taught in martial arts classes and absorbed through our culture.

Couple things first...

PREFACE: THE TRUTH ABOUT ME

I get paid (and paid well) to go into a situation, usually alone and usually outnumbered by sixty or more criminals, and maintain order. I prevent them from preying on each other or attacking officers. That's the job. Now, since I don't fight every day, or even every week (anymore—I'm a sergeant now, one step behind the front line) most of the minutes and hours of the job are pretty easy, far too easy for what they are paying me. But every once in a while on a really, really ugly night, I more than earn my keep.

The fighting happens less, partially from moving up in rank, but even more from the fact that almost every criminal in the area knows me, and I've become better at talking. At CNT training (Crisis Negotiation Team—sometimes called Hostage Negotiators), Cecil, one of the instructors, recommended reading books on salesmanship. In the intro to one book, the author stated that everyone, every single person in the world is engaged in selling *something*—no matter if you were building a car in a factory, performing medicine or changing oil.

I thought, "Bullshit. I'm a jail guard. I'm not selling jack."

Shortly after, there was an extremely stupid and crazy old man who very much wanted to fight five times his weight in officers. It took about twenty minutes to talk him into going along with the process. It was then that I realized I am selling something, a product called "not getting your ass beat" which is very hard to sell to some people.

Here's the resume and *bona fides*. Feel free to skip it.

I enjoy teaching people who have already trained in martial arts how to apply their skills to real conflict. I like teaching officers—people who might need it—the simple, practical skills they need to stay alive or the equally simple and practical skills they need to restrain a threat without getting sued...and I like teaching the difference.

I have a BS degree in experimental psychology with a minor in biology from Oregon State. I'd planned on a double major, but Biochem killed me. While at OSU, I earned varsities in Judo and Fencing, and dabbled in Karate, Tae Kwon Do, and European weapons.

I've studied martial arts since 1981. I've been a corrections officer since 1991. As of this writing, that's fourteen years, twelve of them concentrated in Maximum Security and Booking. In 1998, a lot of things happened. I earned my teaching certificate in *Sosuishitsu-ryu* Jujutsu; I published two articles in national magazines; I was named to the CERT (Corrections Emergency Response Team) and was made the DT and Hand-to-Hand instructor for the team. I was also promoted to sergeant. By the end of the year I was designing and teaching classes for the rest of the agency, both corrections and enforcement. I've been the CERT leader since 2002.

CERT has been a huge force in my life and career. By 1998, I already had lots of "dirt time" in Booking, something over two hundred uses of force, some ugly (PCP and/or outnumbered and/or ambushed and/or weapons), but I'd only had to take care of myself. Suddenly I was responsible for teaching rookies how to do what I did. I had to really think about what made things work.

CERT also allowed me access to huge amounts of training—I'm currently certified with distraction devices (flash-bang grenades), a wide variety of less-lethal technology (40 mm and 37 mm grenade launchers used to fire everything from gas to rubber balls; paintball guns that fire pellets filled with pepper spray; a variety of chemical munitions and shotgun-fired impact devices; pepper spray; and electrical stun devices). I've had the opportunity for specialized high-risk transport EVOC (Emergency Vehicle Operations Course) and have trained with the local U.S. Marshals in close-combat handgun skills. More importantly, I've had the opportunity to use some of these tools and learn what was left out of class. There has been other agency training as well—I've done CNT classes, though a CERT leader won't be in that role; been through the introductory Weapons of Mass Destruction class from FEMA; attended school for the Incident Command System; been certified as a Use of Force and Confrontational Simulation instructor, and recently received a certification as a "Challenge Course Facilitator" in case anyone wants to walk a high wire and do some team building. When I'm not on swing shift, I'm an advisor for the Search and Rescue unit. Swing shift or not, I'm a peer counselor for my deputies.

I was a medic, NBC defense instructor, and rappel master in the

National Guard; studied EMT I and II a long time ago; bounced in a casino for a couple of years; and attended Tom Brown's survival and tracking basic course...and I grew up in the eastern Oregon desert without electricity or running water.

That's just a list. Here's the truth:

Violence is bigger than me. There's more out there and more kinds of violence than I'll ever see...and certainly more than I could survive. I've never been a victim of domestic violence and I've never been taken hostage, but in this book I will presume to give advice on those two subjects. I've never been in an active war zone or a fire fight. Never been bombed, nuked, or gassed—except by trainers.

Violence is a bigger subject than any person will ever understand completely or deeply. I've put as much personal experience into this as I can, along with advice from people I know and trust to be experienced. I've also quoted or paraphrased researchers (many of whom have never bled or spilled blood in either fear or anger) when the research sounded right.

In the end, this is only a book. My goal in writing it is to give my insights to you through the written word. It will be hard to write because survival is very much a matter of guts and feelings and smells and sounds and very, very little a subject of words.

Take my advice for what it is worth. Use what you can use. Discard anything that doesn't make sense.

You don't know me; you've never seen me. For all the *facts* you have, I might be a 400-pound quadriplegic or a seventy year old retiree with delusions. Take the information in this book and treat it skeptically as hell.

Never, ever, ever delegate responsibility for your own safety.

Never, ever, ever override your own experience and common sense on the say-so of some self-appointed "expert."

Never, ever, ever ignore what your eyes see because it isn't what you imagined. And strive to always know the difference between what your eyes are seeing and what your brain is adding.

The format of this book. This book is divided into chapters. The first section, the Introduction, gives a brief overview of what the book is about, who I am, and why I wrote it. You've already either read it or skipped it. Fair enough.

Chapter 1: The Matrix, is an attempt to clear up the language of violence. It addresses the many types of violence, especially how different they can be and how the lessons from one type do not apply to the needs of another.

Chapter 2: How to Think, addresses assumptions about violence, about training, and introduces training for strategy and tactics.

Chapter 3: Violence, describes the dynamics of violence. It is focused on criminal violence—how it happens and what it is like. It will also cover the affects of adrenaline and stress hormones that accompany a sudden attack and how to deal with them.

Chapter 4: Predators, is about criminals—who they are, how they think and act. What you can expect from them, and what knowledge is not important in a moment of crisis.

Chapter 5: Training, will give advice and drills to help adapt your training to the realities of violence.

Chapter 6: Making Physical Defense Work, is about physical response to violence—not about effective technique but about what makes a technique effective.

Chapter 7: After, discusses the after-effects of violence—what to expect and how to deal with the psychological effects of either surviving a sudden assault or long-term exposure to a violent environment.

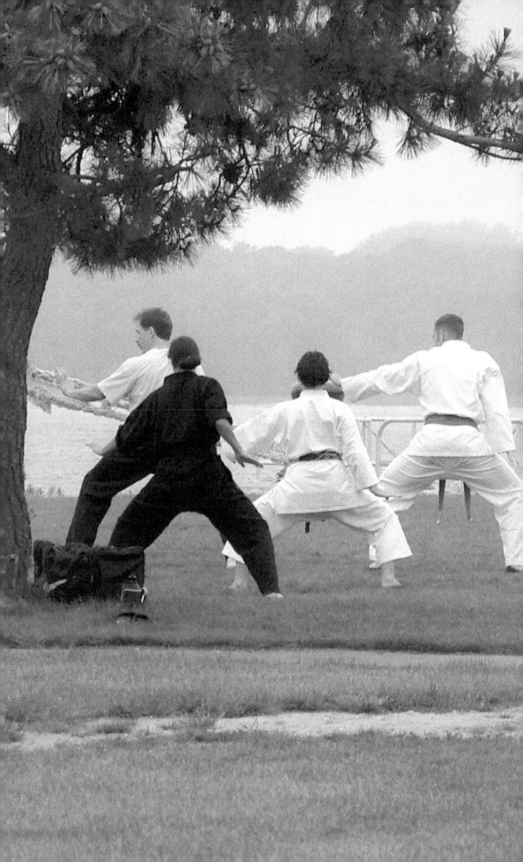

CHAPTER 1: THE MATRIX

You all know the story of the blind men and the elephant, right? It was originally published in a poem by John Godfrey Saxe that was about the silliness of humans disputing the nature of gods and religions.

The blind men, each very famous for wisdom and intelligence, walk up to an elephant, touch a piece, and begin to explain and describe the entire animal. The first touches the elephant's side and declares that an elephant is just like a wall. The second, happening to grab hold of a tusk, knows that an elephant is just like a spear (okay, dull and curved and too thick but otherwise *exactly* like a spear...I don't think this was the smartest of the blind men). From his short experience with the trunk, the third decides that an elephant is just like a snake

I don't need to go on, do I?

Not to hit you over the head with the animal metaphors, but violence is a big animal and many people who have seen only a part of it are more than willing to sell you their expertise. Does someone who has been in a few bar brawls really know any more about violence than the guy who grabbed the elephant's ear knows about elephants? Bar brawling experience *is* real and it is exactly what it is, but it won't help you or even provide much insight into military operations or rape survival.

A truly devious mind that understands the principles can occasionally generalize from one type of conflict, say flying a combat mission, to very different types of conflict, such as crime prevention, debate or tactical assault. But that skill is both rare and limited. No matter how good you are at generalizing, there is a point where it doesn't work and you descend into philosophy at the cost of survival.

Many martial arts, martial artists, and even people who fight for real on a regular basis have also only seen a very small part of this very big thing. Often, the best know one aspect very well, but that is only one aspect.

Some of the experts who are willing to sell you their insights have never seen a real elephant. Many people, almost all men in my

1

Group *kata* at Cape Cod
Courtesy Kamila Z. Miller

experience, are willing to talk at length on the subjects of fighting and violence. They will lecture, expound, and debate.

Know this: Watching every martial arts movie ever filmed gives you as much understanding of fighting as a child watching *Dumbo* learned about elephants. Learning a martial art often teaches you as much as a taxidermist would know about elephants. Watching boxing or the UFC teaches as much as a trip to the zoo or the circus. Really, really studying the best research available gives you an incredible amount of knowledge about violence or about elephants, but there is always one detail missing.

When you are standing next to an elephant, it is huge. It could crush you at will or tear you in half, and there is nothing you could do. The advantage of being blind, of only knowing a part of this beast, is the comfortable illusion of safety.

section 1.1: the tactical matrix—an example

Violence isn't just a big animal. It is complicated as hell. If you ever really wanted to get a handle on just one piece—interpersonal violence—you would need to understand physics, anatomy and physiology, athletics, criminal law, group dynamics, criminal dynamics, evolutionary psychology, biology and evolutionary biology, endocrinology, strategy, and even moral philosophy. In this great big complex mess, if you want to survive, you need a quick and simple answer. That's hard.

A matrix is used to describe and analyze a multidimensional event in a multidimensional way. Ask a martial artist, "What's your favorite attack?" or "What's your favorite combination?" and they will have an answer. For a few years, mine was a backfist/sidekick combination. Remember that. It will come up in a few paragraphs.

There are many ways to break things up. Consider this as one example. There are four different ways that a fight can arise:

(1) You are completely surprised, hit before you are aware that a conflict has arisen.
(2) You felt something was going on but weren't sure what.
(3) You knew it was coming and you were ready, a mutual combat.
(4) You ambushed the other guy, initiating action when he was completely surprised.

There are also three different levels of force that you can use. (A) You must not injure the other person, (e.g. getting the car keys from drunken Uncle Bob). (B) It's okay to injure, but not to kill. (C) Killing is both legally justified and prudent.

This makes a simple 3x4 matrix of twelve options:

Figure 1.1: The Tactical Matrix

	SURPRISED	ALERTED	MUTUAL	ATTACKING
NO INJURY				
INJURY				
LETHAL				

In only one of these twelve possible scenarios is the backfist/sidekick a really good option. It is workable in perhaps two more, but for seventy-five percent of the options, my "favorite" technique is worthless.

You can plug almost any technique, tactic, or even system into the matrix and see where it applies. Karate's core strategy is to "do damage"—close in and hit hard. Given that it is difficult (not impossible) to kill with a bare hand, where does Karate fit on the matrix? Where does boxing fit? Sword and shield? Where does a handgun fit? Can you use a handgun when you are completely surprised?

	SURPRISED	ALERTED	MUTUAL	ATTACKING
NO INJURY	Inappropriate due to risk of injury/ requires time and distance	Inappropriate due to risk of injury	Inappropriate due to risk of injury	Inappropriate due to risk of injury
INJURY	Requires some time and distance. Won't work	Possible, if attacker gives time	Good	Possible, but feint is inefficient if you have surprise
LETHAL	Insufficient force, time, and distance. Unworkable	Insufficient force	Insufficient force	Insufficient force

Using a backfist/sidekick combination in an
example of a simple tactical matrix.

	SURPRISED	ALERTED	MUTUAL	ATTACKING
NO INJURY	Inappropriate due to risk of fatality/no time to draw	Inappropriate due to risk of fatality	Inappropriate due to risk of fatality	Inappropriate due to risk of fatality
INJURY	Risk of fatality/ no time to draw	Risk of fatality	Risk of fatality	Risk of fatality
LETHAL	Possible, if you can overcome surprise and draw weapon	Effective	Effective	Effective

Using a firearm as an example.

Looking at it like that, however, is a fundamental flaw in thinking. To work from technique to situation is backwards. The parameters, in this case "level of surprise" and "acceptable damage," dictate the matrix. Each box in the matrix represents a type of situation. To go through life being very skilled at one or two aspects of the matrix, and hoping the violence you run into will happen to match your boxes, is dangerous and yet very common.

Here's a rule for life: You don't get to pick what kinds of bad things will happen to you. You may prepare all your life to take on a cannibalistic knife-wielding sociopath. You may get stuck with a soccer riot. Or a road rage incident with a semi. Or a pickup full of baseball bat swinging drunks. Or nothing at all. You don't get to choose.

The purpose of the tactical matrix is to introduce regular people to the idea that violence is complex. For martial artists, it is important to understand that preparing for one thing is not preparing for all things. For citizens watching the news, trying to figure out if what an officer did was the right thing, it's important to understand that not everything can be solved with a wristlock or a few kind words. Violence is complex.

The tactical matrix here is NOT an answer or a guide. It is an example. It's not even an example of types of fights. It is a first step in demonstrating complexity. The matrix can be extended infinitely. Multiple bad guys? Three ways that can break down—my side outnumbers you, your side outnumbers me or we're even. The matrix now has 36 boxes. Weapons? I have a weapon, you have a weapon, we both do or neither of us do. Four options and the matrix jumps to 144 boxes.

Got it? Good, 'cause now we're going to get complicated.

section 1.2: the strategic matrix: what martial arts tries to be

A *New York Times* article dated June 7, 2005 describes a video of an officer in a traffic stop taking fire from the driver and his partner running away. The officer who ran away chose the perfect option for self-defense. It was not the best option for his partner. It was not what he was trained and expected to do. He was trained and expected to engage the threat.

Officers on patrol avoid hand-to-hand encounters. Fights are dangerous. Even when you win, there is a possibility of injury, exposure to blood-borne pathogens such as HIV and hepatitis, or a lawsuit. Within that context, there are two distinctive hand-to-hand skills that an officer needs. In the ugly, surprise situation, taking damage and unprepared, the officer needs brutal close-quarters survival skills. Putting handcuffs on an unruly drunk who doesn't want to go to jail but doesn't really want to hurt you requires different skills, different techniques, and a different mindset.

Sometimes there are more. A SWAT sniper needs a crystal clear thought process and the ability to deal with hours of boredom and discomfort. The point man on an entry team doesn't need or use the same techniques or mindset as the sniper, isn't interested in semi-compliant handcuffing and damn well better not be surprised if he works for me. He is the "surprisor."

In just one profession, four different skill sets for dealing with physical conflict. Not one of them is like dueling, sparring, or waging a war.

Martial arts try to do more than that. Some studios promise self-defense skills and tournament trophies, discipline and self-discovery, fitness and confidence, and even spiritual growth and enlightenment.

How well do these goals really mesh?

Cardiovascular fitness is extremely important for health and longevity and should be the cornerstone of any fitness regimen, yet fighting for your life is profoundly anaerobic. Whether you had a good breakfast will have a greater effect on your endurance thirty seconds into the fight (and thirty seconds is a long time in an ambush) than your ability to run a marathon.

Spiritual growth, the measure of many modern martial arts, is a difficult concept to pin down. I once asked my *sensei* in Jujutsu if there was a spiritual discipline associated with *Sosuishitsu-ryu*. Dave said, "Oh. Sure. The dead guy doesn't get to go to church. Don't try to read too much into this, Rory. It's not a way of life. It's a collection of skills a samurai might need if he wanted to go home to his family."

Martial arts and martial artists often try to do it all. They teach self-defense and sparring and streetfighting and fitness and personal development, as if they were the same thing. They aren't even related.

Very, very different things get lumped under the general heading of "violence." Two boxers in a contest of strategy, strength, skill, and will. A drunken husband beating his wife. Two highschoolers punch-

	SELF-DEFENSE	DUEL	SPORT	COMBAT	ASSAULT	SPIRITUAL GROWTH	FITNESS
REALITY OF EVENT	Recovery from bad luck or stupidity	Glorified Monkey Dance	Contest of the similar	Monkey Dance between groups	Neutralize threat/enemy	Mostly stumbling in the dark	Physical training
REALITY TO PERSON	Absolute threat to health, survival, and identity	Voluntary physical danger for social gain	Test of self	Boredom, confusion, busywork, and occasional terror	Job	Reality doesn't go here	Part of life
REAL GOAL	Survive	Maintain or increase social standing	Ego validation	Please supervisors and peers	Mission and survive	Achieve and maintain *satori*	Varies, improve appearance
BEST GOAL	Prevent, if too late, escape	Win with style	Prove/test oneself	Defeat opposing group, preferably by display	Mission and survive	Understand self	Improve health
DISTRACTERS Fake Goals; Illusions	Maintain social illusions; deny reality	No choice	Fear of losing; belief that X=Y	Personal meaning or mission, freelancing	Fear of liability, crusade, ego, admin interference	Understand the world, ego	Appearance equals ability
OPTIMAL MINDSET	None or rage	Arrogance w/o overconfidence	Athletic focus, "the zone"	Obedience	Implacable predator	Perceive	Everyday—habit
BEST ASSET	Aggressive reactions	Cunning?	Skill? Cunning?	Teamwork and discipline	Planning and preparation	Bullshit detector (or openness)	Perseverance
STRATEGY	Beat the freeze	Dazzle the opponent	Psych the opponent out	Control individuality, make troops predictable	Shock and Awe	Listen, watch, feel	Stick to training plan
TRAINING FOCUS	Contact response	Skill, fitness, and conventions; showmanship	Skill and fitness	Obedience and rote specific skills	Teamwork, skills, threat analysis	Letting distractions go	Training, nutrition, recuperation
REAL DANGER	Loss of life, identity	Death	Injury	Stupid leaders	Luck	Being defrauded: otherwise, very safe	Overtraining, training for wrong thing
PERCEIVED DANGER	Same	Dishonor, loss of face, embarrassment	Damage to identity	Enemy	Enemy	Inability to see the world "in light"	None

Matrix of Martial Arts and Violence: Differences of Type

ing it out in the parking lot. A mental health professional trying to hold down a schizophrenic so that a sedative can be administered. An officer walking into a robbery in progress finds himself in a shoot-out. Soldiers entering a building in hostile territory. A rapist pushing in the partially open door of an apartment. An entry team preparing to serve a search warrant on a drug house with armed suspects. A Victorian era duel with small swords.

Because they involve people in conflict and people get hurt, we lump them together as violence, but they aren't the same and the skills and mindset from one situation don't carry over automatically to the other.

Self-defense is clearly my focus in this book. What is it? It is recovery from stupidity or bad luck, from finding yourself in a position you would have given almost anything to prevent. It is difficult to train for because of the surprise element and because you may be injured before you are aware of the conflict. The critical element is to overcome the shock and surprise so that you can act, to "beat the freeze." Self-defense is about *recovery*. The ideal is to prevent the situation. The optimal mindset is often a conditioned response that requires no thought (for the first half-second of the attack) or a focused rage.

The *duel* is out of fashion in our day and age. It was (and occasionally is) a glorified Monkey Dance (*See* Section 3.1) forced by society. It was a contest to see who could better uphold the standards of the day, thus it was fought over insults and unacceptable behavior and not more material injury. It was possibly more about show than survival. There was a "right" way to win. This still happens in rare incidents of "*dojo arashi*" when martial artists go to other martial arts schools to challenge the instructors. The early UFC bouts also tried to take on this element in the "style versus style" but they were very different.

Can we use the skills, mindset, and strategies of the duel in a self-defense situation?

Sport is a contest between two people; different than the duel because it is something the practitioners seek and not something they feel they must do to preserve their place in society. It is admirable, to me, because the real goal is to test yourself. For most, it's not about domination but about what they have, what they can do, what they've learned. Mixed martial arts (MMA) is part of a long evolution of taking this concept as far as it can go safely.

Is the righteous rage, which has gotten so many people through an attempted rape, an efficient emotional response for a high school wrestling match?

By *combat*, I specifically mean war. Combat is a very different experience for generals than for soldiers. Generals can look at percentage killed, take risks, sacrifice, and maneuver men. For the generals, there are acceptable losses and you can continue to fight if you suffer twenty percent killed. For the soldier, it is binary: You are alive or you are dead. Generals win wars. Teams win wars. I remember my drill sergeant yelling, "You are not an individual! You are a part of this team!" In order for the generals to win, the soldiers must be predictable. The general has to be certain that if he orders them to march or attack or hold position, they will. Thus, obedience is critical and it is enforced by a culture that will do what is expected because they don't want to let the rest of the team down.

Given that the most common lead up to an attack on a woman is to show a weapon and order her to obey, is being trained to obey, whether in the military or one of the militaristic *dojos,* a good training method for self-defense?

Assault isn't just for criminals. Elite military teams, hostage rescue, SWAT, and entry teams use this mindset as much as criminals do. They don't want to be tested or find out what their limitations are, they want to get the job done and go home. The mindset is implacable and predatory. They use surprise, superior numbers, and superior weapons—every cheat they can, and they practice. On the rare, rare occasions when my team made a fast entry and someone actually fought, the only emotion that I registered was that I was *offended* that they resisted, and we rolled right over the threat(s) like a force of nature.

If you can truly flip the switch from surprised, overwhelmed, and terrified to the assault mindset, I can't teach you much. This is the opposite of the "frozen" response often triggered by a sudden assault, and we train hard to trigger that freeze in others.

Spiritual growth is very difficult to define. If it is a depth of understanding of the human condition, you will grow more by living and serving and talking to people than you will ever learn in a class of any kind. If it is understanding of yourself, you will learn the most by challenging your fears and dislikes, and few people stick with a class that they fear and dislike. If it is a happy feeling that all is right with the world and there is a plan and everything is wonderful and good...you can get it from heroin cheaper and faster. If it is something great and magical that will open up your psychic powers, keep playing video games. There is a danger here that I don't properly address in the simple matrix and is beyond the scope of this book: people want to believe in magic and secrets and there are other people who will satisfy those beliefs for money or power. This can result in abuse and trauma, the very opposite of self-defense.

Fitness is objectively the most important effect of martial arts training. The physical skills and self-defense aspects of training will never save as many people from violence as the conditioning will save from early heart attacks. If you study Judo, Jujutsu, or Aikido, you will probably never use the skills to throw an attacker, but I can almost guarantee that you will and have used the breakfalls to prevent injury. Properly trained, many martial arts give balanced development of muscle, strength and aerobic training, increases in flexibility and agility, and all at a relatively low risk of injury. It may not be as efficient as a good circuit program in these areas, but it can be more fun and you will stick with the exercise program that you enjoy.

Fitness will never hurt you in a self-defense situation. Even aerobic conditioning, which rarely activates in a fight, will help to dissipate the stress hormones that will affect your mind and body. When comparing fitness with self-defense, the problems come from the other direction. Self-defense is largely about dealing with surprise and fear and pain, none of which is useful in developing fitness.

One example from the other dimension of the matrix to hammer home the point: Look at the optimum mindset for each of the examples of conflict.

The implacable predatory mindset of the assault is powerful. It is cold-blooded, calculating, and utterly controlled. It is also inhuman, reducing the target of the assault from human to either a resource (in the criminal mind) or a threat (in the mind of an entry team).

This mindset, in my experience, horrifies the people seeking spiritual growth. It is a natural mindset and beautiful in its place, but it is scary to someone who is seeking light and love and harmony. People who imagine the harmony of nature are often willfully blind to the savagery between wolf and rabbit. The assault mindset can revel in that savagery.

The assault mindset in a sporting competition is completely unacceptable. From the assault mindset, if you are scheduled to fight a world champion heavyweight boxer on Thursday, you shoot him on Tuesday. It is not just beyond cheating—cheating has no meaning in the mind of a predator—there are only odds, tactics, and meat. This comparison is doubly true for the duel.

Some elite elements in combat develop the predator mindset. It requires trust and respect to get an entire team into that mindset. Far more teams fake it by hard training under a good leader than actually have the mindset. True predators are unpredictable and that makes the chain of command uncomfortable. They will get the job done but will ignore any parameter or rule of engagement set by command that does not seem important to them. Because of this, they are idolized in times of serious conflict and marginalized, ignored, or pushed aside when combat is rare.

Fitness training is about your self. There is no prey and therefore nothing for the predator mindset to focus on. A predator without prey is a fat, lazy cat that likes to play and eat and sleep.

The predator mindset is a choice. No one is in that mind at all times—it has too many blind spots to function in normal society. Self-defense is never a choice. The attacker is in the predator mindset, not the victim. The victim will have to deal with shock and total surprise, the predator won't. The essence of self-defense is breaking out of the

11

frozen mindset you have been shocked into. If you can access the predator mindset a few seconds into the attack, you can turn the attack into something else. That's powerful, but takes great experience.

This matrix could be extended almost infinitely in either dimension. Fight choreography for films, stuntwork, performing arts, and restraining mental patients without injuring them could all be added across the top. Timing differences, best class of techniques, ideal opponent, and reliance on technology could all have a space.

Despite the wide variety of skills and complete incompatibility of the mindsets or strategy, martial artists are often convinced that they are training for all of these things simultaneously. In strictly regimented classes where things are done by rote and without question, you can see the military roots of a soldier's art...but that obedient mindset can set students up for failure if they are victimized by an authority figure or overwhelmed by an attacker who uses verbal commands with his assault. Some instructors extol the virtues of the predatory mindset, the "eyes of a tiger," without teaching how to get there from a moment of surprise, pain, and fear (for self-defense) or dealing with the logical consequences for sport—a true predator cheats in profound ways. Not the little ways, like illegal nerve gouges in the grapple, but big ways like getting a bunch of friends and weapons and finishing the fight in the locker room before the match starts.

This extends well beyond martial arts and into the world of conflict and the perception of conflict in general. In the world of movies, boots and fists and guns are used interchangeably. In real life, the skills, needs, and legal justification for striking and shooting are very different.

Police solutions to military problems are doomed to fail just as military solutions to police problems will never be allowed in a free society.

You will bring your experience and training (your touch of the elephant) to bear whenever you read about a military operation or see a story about a police shooting on the news.

Remember this—that the fair play and good sportsmanship you learned as a child were predicated on two fairly matched people who wanted to be there, not some drugged-up freak with a knife and an officer answering a call.

That on TV and in your martial arts classes, they make it look easy to take away a knife—an officer knows that if someone is within seven yards he can be stabbed more than once before he can even draw his weapon.

That in the movies, the sniper can coolly make head shot after head shot at five hundred yards, protecting his team. In real life, snipers have tried in vain to identify a target through smoke and muzzle flash as civilians get slaughtered.

That in books, the radios always seem to work, cell phones never go off when you are trying to get into a position, the good guy always carries enough ammo, and no one ever just bleeds out and dies from a "flesh wound."

That when the newspaper decries the brutality of the officer who used force on a fifteen-year-old, mentally-ill "child," all the officer saw was a 280 pound person in an altered mental state coming at him, swinging a club.

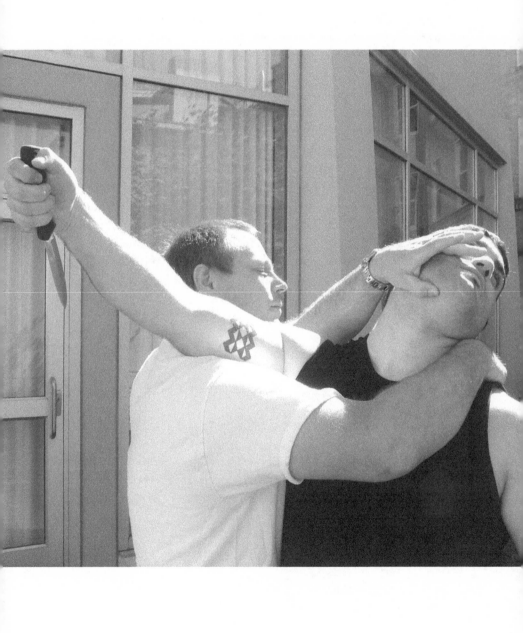

CHAPTER 2: HOW TO THINK

section 2.1: assumptions and epistemology

Before we start explaining strategy or tactics, we need to address assumptions. Assumptions are those things you believe to be true without really considering them. They provide the background for much of how you see the parts of the world that you have never experienced. For instance, you can *assume* that people elsewhere in the world are very similar to the people you know, or you can *assume* that they are very different. Either point of view will color all of your interactions with and perceptions of those people. Like many things, your assumptions affect you far more than they affect the world.

The world is a big place and full of many things. We could not function if we had to deal with each event in our life as a new and separate thing. We will start the car tomorrow the way that we started it yesterday. When we buy a new car, it will start and operate very much like the old one. Assumptions, in a large part of our daily life, are necessary and usually harmless.

We get into trouble when we base our assumptions on either irrelevant comparison or bad sources. No amount of driving a car will prepare you for riding a bicycle for the first time. No matter how hard you convince yourself that they are both vehicles, both just machines, the skills are different. Cars and bicycles are irrelevant comparisons. A bad source would be taking driving lessons from someone who has never driven a car. Worse would be learning to drive a car from a bicyclist who THINKS it's the same as driving a car.

There is a second condition that must be met before your bad assumptions can harm you. The subject must *matter*. You can believe anything you want about the best way to approach extraterrestrials or how you would broker world peace and since it will never be tested, you can believe anything you want with no consequences. Martial arts

The author gouging Luke while praticing no-hands elbow control.
Courtesy Kamila Z. Miller

and self-defense are tricky, because for most practitioners whether they work or not will never really matter. It will never be tested. They can learn and believe and teach any foolishness they want. It will only be a source for interesting conversation.

Then, occasionally it will matter very much to an isolated individual. The stakes are high.

It is very difficult to analyze your own assumptions. In your own mind, they are only "the things you believe," the "true" things. As I wrote above, they are the things you never really considered...because you've never really doubted them.

Epistemology is the study of how people and societies decide what is true. What is your personal epistemology? What sources do you consider unimpeachable? If it's on the eleven o'clock news, does that make it true? If all your friends are saying something, does that make it true? If it's in *Science Digest* or *Scientific American*, do you believe it? If your pastor said it, is it gospel? (sorry, pun) Do you trust your personal experience?

Personal experience would seem to be a no-brainer but very, very few people will trust their own experience against the word of either many people or a single "expert."

One of my co-workers is amazing. He's a hell of a nice guy and hell itself in a fight—huge, strong, and not completely sane. We were taking a course in a personal protection system and the instructor was describing a "Straightblast" technique where you applied chained punches to the face with aggressive forward movement. The instructor was very good, a very charismatic young man who had been training for years but didn't have a lot of experience in our environment.

The instructor explained how under a Straightblast the threat will retreat. My friend said, "But what if he doesn't? What if he steps in?"

I thought, "Brother, the last guy who moved in on you and STABBED you, you lifted him up in the air and slammed him down so hard you broke his spine! Why the hell are you listening to this guy when you have more experience than him and everyone he knows combined?"

But my friend, this truly awesome survival fighter, had completely set aside his own experience...because this instructor was an "expert."

Even when you develop a belief based on personal experience, you are influenced in subtle ways. Rarely, if ever, is personal experience the sole basis of a belief. As an example, most people believe that the sun will rise tomorrow. If you questioned them, a good percentage of them will say that this belief is based on personal experience. It seems reasonable to believe that if the sun has risen every day of your life, it will continue to do so forever.

However, since the same people have awakened every morning to observe this have also awakened, isn't it equally reasonable to believe that since you have woken up every day of your life you will continue to do so forever? Yet, very few people think that they are immortal. My wife says, "We're immortal, so far."

The best advice in this book will serve to enrich your life more than it will contribute to your survival. This is one of those bits. Examine your own epistemology. Look at your beliefs, and the source of those beliefs. Some of your beliefs came from early training or bad sources. Some of your sources were chosen because you knew they supported your preexisting point of view. Look very deeply at those sources that you accept without question.

As you do this, it will allow you to see many things that you have thought of as true as merely opinions, and give you great freedom in exploring and understanding both your world and other people's.

Because of the nature of this book, I want you to apply this concept first to violence. Violence, for most of us, is unknown territory. Though martial artists have studied "fighting," and everyone has been raised in a culture where stylized violence is everywhere, very little of what we know is based on experience, and very much is based on word of mouth. It is, for many people, *entirely* assumption. If the source of information is good, the martial artist may be able to defend him or herself with the skills. If the source is bad, the skills taught can actually decrease survivability.

I want to be very clear here. What you have trained in and been taught is "word of mouth." Until you do it yourself, for real, you can't evaluate it with accuracy. Experience in the *dojo* is experience in the *dojo*. Experience in the ring is experience in the ring. Experience on the street is experience on the street. There is some overlap in skills; some lessons transfer. But a black belt in Judo will teach you as much about sudden assault as being mugged will teach you about Judo. And my experience will always be your word of mouth.

You have certain assumptions about what conflict is like. If you are interested in self-defense, you will choose a martial art based on its similarity to your assumptions. As you read books or listen to TV analysis of crimes and war, you will subtly pick your sources to mirror your views. In some cases, if the student isn't careful or becomes enamored of the system or instructor, he will ignore real experience if it doesn't match his assumption.

John has studied two martial arts and has been in several "encounters." He considers one of his martial arts unrealistic and worthless, largely because he fights "so much harder" sparring in his new grappling system. Yet, studying his old, "worthless" style, he was surprised and responded with (of all things) a kick to the chin. The threat was taken down in under a second with no harm to John. After studying his new style for some time, he chose to interfere in a conflict between a biker and someone who owed the biker money. John got stomped pretty bad. He feels it would have been much worse if he had stuck with his original martial art.

Despite his own experience of a perfect fight (one move, complete takeout) and a bad one, John likes his new art because the sparring feels more like he imagines a fight should feel. It matches his assumptions and, like many people, his assumptions override reality.

If you study a formal martial art, there is another set of assumptions that you must deal with: the assumptions of your style. The first major assumption is a belief in what a "fight" is and looks like. The second is what defines a "win." For the old style of Jujutsu that I study, the assumed opponent was an armed and armored warrior, the assumed environment was a battlefield full of armed people, the assumed situation was that your weapon had been dropped or broken suddenly, and the assumed goal was to get an opponent's weapon, probably by killing him. This list of assumptions drives almost everything in the style. It forces a close, brutal, quick, and aggressive concept based entirely on gross motor skills.

Most styles and instructors are remarkably well adapted to getting the win in the right kind of fight, and crippled when the fight doesn't match their expectation or when the conditions of a win change.

Every style is for *something*, a collection of tactics and tools to deal with what the founder was afraid of. A style based on the founder's fear of losing a non-contact tournament will look different, even if it is just as well-adapted for that idea of a fight as my Jujutsu is for its time and place.

Understand thoroughly what your style is for. Violence is a very broad category of human interaction. Many, many instructors attempt to apply something designed for a very narrow aspect of violence, such as unarmed dueling, and extrapolate it to other incompatible areas, such as ambush survival. My Jujutsu, for instance, is wonderfully adapted to close-range medieval battlefield emergencies. From there it is a fairly easy stretch to predatory assault survival, but difficult to adapt to either sparring or the pain-compliance/restraint level of police Defensive Tactics (DTs).

Each instructor also has assumptions based on his or her experience, training, and (too often) television and popular culture.

At a seminar, I met a martial arts instructor of great skill in his specialty—under the right circumstances, he could dodge and send people sailing with very little effort. It bothered me, because the operative concept was "under the right circumstances." If someone rushed him from at least two long paces away and flinched past their own point of balance, his techniques would work. Otherwise, not so well. They didn't work, generally, on the other instructors there, and he had brought his own student so that he could demonstrate successfully.

I don't think this was conscious. I met the instructor and talked with him. I genuinely liked and respected him. I believe that in his own mind, his techniques did work on the other instructors. If they didn't, he attributed it to our vast skill. I don't think for a second that he realized that he had taught his student to flinch in a certain way so that the techniques would work.

The two long paces bothered me more, because he espoused that attacks happen exclusively at that range, and they don't. He set me at that distance and asked how I would attack. I smiled, walked up, put an arm around his shoulders, and fired a knee into his thigh. He laughed and said, "I'd never let you get that close." He just had. Without a beat, he turned back to the lesson.

He had superb skill and he (or his instructors) had rewritten the map of the world so that the techniques would work. Since the techniques required two paces, attacks must come at two paces, right? Otherwise, the techniques would have been designed differently. Right?

Imagine studying something for a decade or more that you will never actually use. You have worked to perfect it, but without a touchstone to reality, how do you know what perfection looks like?

He told me about a serious assault he had been subjected to—it was bloody and messy, an ambush at close quarters with lumber and boots. It didn't happen at two paces, or from the front. The two he could see were closer than he believes he would ever let anyone get, and he didn't see the third.

I assume that sometime after this incident he found his martial art, fell in love with it, and found great comfort and a feeling of safety in its practice. Does he ever think about that attack within the context of what he teaches? How do illusions become so powerful that they seem more real and affect beliefs more than an event as horrific as the one he experienced?

The assumptions of his style and his respect for them were able to outweigh a brutal and critical personal experience. That is powerful and very, very dangerous.

section 2.2: the power of assumption

Some of our assumptions are so closely held that we will cling to them, even in the face of overwhelming evidence. Many, many people discount their own experience as an "aberration," preferring to trust in "common sense" or tradition or the word of an "expert."

I've caught myself doing this.

I've had five real encounters with knife-wielding threats...sort of.

The first was downward stab at my shoulder from a teenage girl that I blocked and armlocked easily. So that doesn't count, right? It was too easy, not the scary and desperate situation I've trained for—and it was "only a girl" and only a pair of scissors.

The second was a straight-up assassination attempt. A somewhat unbalanced relative tried with all her might and speed to put a steak knife in my kidney from behind. I'm only alive because I saw a reflection and my body acted immediately and explosively. Was it a "real knife defense" if I am aware that I'm only alive because of luck?

The third was in a casino in Reno. I was ordering a bum who had been stealing credits from other customers to leave, and he pulled a knife. I stayed calm, hands up, and continued moving towards him, keeping my voice calm. I knew that my legs were slightly longer than his weapon range and I was fully prepared to kick as soon as the critical distance was reached—it wasn't going to be a friendly sparring kick, either. I was going for a forty-yard punt. With each step forward that I took, he took one backwards until he was out of the casino. It never went to combat. Does it count?

The fourth was searching a fresh arrestee in booking. He was a little drunk, his cuffs were off, and he had his hands on the counter facing away from me for the pat search. At the base of his spine there was a roughly cylindrical object under his shirt. I thought "knife!" at first, but when I asked him what it was, he said, "Let me show you!" and he spun, reaching under the shirt exactly the same way I'd practiced to draw my weapon from under my jacket. He never got it out. Knife or gun, I didn't know and didn't care. I hit him as hard and fast as I've ever hit a human being, driving his head into the wall, the counter, and sweeping his legs out from under him. His head hit

21

three hard surfaces—wall, counter, and floor—in about a second. If he never got a chance to draw, was it really weapons defense? If I thought it was a knife and it was only a cigarette lighter, does it count?

The last should have been ugly. A freak on PCP was placed in an isolation cell in Reception. With his fingers, he pulled six concrete screws out of the wall to get access to the stainless steel mirror. He then broke the steel mirror in half so that he would have one shank in each hand. On-duty staff sprayed him with five large canisters of pepper spray and he didn't even shut his eyes. So they called us, CERT (Corrections Emergency Response Team). We handled it without a problem. Does it count as knife defense if I was dealing with it as part of a specially trained and equipped eight-man team?

These are all real encounters. Any of them could have ended my life. But because they don't fit my assumptions, because they don't look like the picture I have in my head of a "knife fight," I sometimes downplay the lessons I learned, and this is a danger. Lessons from life are gifts and they should not be ignored.

One of the reasons that it is hard to find an experienced instructor for real violence is that it is hard to survive enough encounters to learn what worked and what didn't. As odd and weak as I sometimes see these experiences, how many "experts" in bladed weapon defense have had five or more encounters? Five is a very large number in this field...but would you train for a kickboxing tournament under a coach who had only five matches? Especially if he freely admitted that of those five he cheated on two, got lucky on one, had one opponent back out, and won the first against an opponent below his weight class? Hell no...but in this field, five is a lot of experience.

Sometimes, it's not only discounting real experience but taking experience from bad sources and labeling it "truth" that can mentally cripple you.

One of my students was concerned that she couldn't hurt a large man. I told her to imagine a two-hundred-pound man holding a small cat. Could the man kill the cat? Sure.

"Now imagine I throw a bucket of water on them. What happens?"

"The cat goes berserk and starts scratching the guy up."

"Does the guy let go?"

"Probably."

"So the cat wins?"

"I guess. Sure."

"So you're telling me that an eight pound cat can hurt a big man and you can't?"

"The cat has claws and teeth."

"And you don't?"

She thought for a minute. "But I've wrestled with my boyfriends before and I couldn't do anything." Aha.

She had taken a situation where she had no desire to cause injury, no fear, probably wanted to strengthen and deepen the relationship, and she had chosen that incident to base her assumptions about combat. Those assumptions nearly made her give up on training.

There are fads in the law enforcement community and we love experts. When the UFC started and the Gracies were winning everything, "Tactical Groundfighting Courses" started springing up all over the country. They were barely-altered aspects of Gracie Jujitsu or wrestling. Many of the classes I saw showed a fundamental ignorance of the job. Sport grappling immobilizes opponents on their backs; LEOs immobilize face down, for handcuffing. Sport grappling takes up space with tight body contact; in law enforcement, at that range the threat can kill us with weapons from our own belts.

The goals of the two are not the same. In many ways it was as if LEOs were attempting to improve their ability to fly fighter jets by taking lessons from the best submariners in the world.

One last story: It is said that when a baby elephant is first trained, a rope or chain is tied around its ankle and it will struggle and pull and fight against the chain. When it learns that it cannot break the chain, the chain can be replaced with a bit of twine and the elephant will never try to break it. The elephant assumes it can't, and so a full-grown elephant can be held by a piece of string.

Many of your assumptions came from childhood. You are no longer a child.

Many came from earlier in your training—you have grown and changed since then.

Many came from unreliable sources. You can make up your own mind.

Do not let yourself be crippled by something that only exists in your mind.

section 2.3: common sources of knowledge about violence

We are, all of us, both teachers and students. As teachers, we give our students information. As students, we learn from our teachers. The teachers give us knowledge. This knowledge came from somewhere, from one of four sources:

- Experience
- Reason
- Tradition
- Entertainment and Recreation

I like experience. It helps to winnow the BS from the truth. It allows you to pass on a little of the mindset, a few of the tricks, some of the obstacles that they will face. It leads to a perspective that is unique. But realistically, how many instructors have enough hands-on experience in real violence to pass anything along? Very few. The instructors who have experienced enough violence to be able to generalize are even more rare.

Additionally, violence is extremely idiosyncratic. I honestly don't know if my experience will match yours. I don't know if our bodies and minds will react in the same way to the cascade of stress hormones. I can't honestly tell you how much of my survival is based on judgment or skill or luck.

I was discussing this with one of my students, explaining that unlike almost anything else, the more experience of violence you have the less sure you are that things will work out. Jordan put it in perspective: "Sounds like a case of the more you know, the more you realize you don't know."

Experience, in my opinion, could not give rise to a new martial art. Given the idiosyncratic nature and the improbability of surviving enough high-end encounters, it would be hard to come up with guiding principles or even a core of reliable techniques. I am painfully aware that things that worked in one instant have failed utterly in others.

Decapitating goats and the limits of reason. When I was very young I read a book called *The Far Arena* by Richard Sapir. The premise of the book was that a Roman gladiator had been frozen in arctic ice and miraculously brought back to life in modern times. One section stuck with me for many years. The gladiator was ruminating on decapitation. He explained that it was rare, that in all his time in the arena he had only seen it done once, by an enormous Germanic barbarian. He explained in great detail about the different layers of tissue, the toughness of the muscle, and how things that cut muscle tend to be poor at cutting bone and vise versa. It made perfect sense. I filed it away in the back of my head and believed, without challenging it, that beheading someone or something would be a very difficult task indeed.

Years later I was asked to help a friend butcher some goats. The first step, of course, was killing the animal. We wanted to minimize pain and panic. Cutting throats can work. A gunshot to the brainstem can work (but the other goats tend to get scared and are harder to control). I'd been practicing with sword for years. Both the owner of the goats and my wife write fiction of the sort where details on beheading might be useful. I volunteered to lop the goats' heads off.

Mary held a rope and the goat pulled against it, stretching its neck nicely. I used the sword my wife had given me for our first anniversary, a single-edged hand-and-a-half forged by Cord. *The Far Arena* firmly in mind, I prepared for a power stroke. All of my skill and all of my power...The sword went through the neck like it wasn't there. In all the animals we butchered that day, I only felt any resistance once—we didn't use the rope and I did a backhand horizontal stroke. That goat died instantly with its spine severed but the blade didn't go all the way through the front of the neck. Later, there is a stage in the butchering process where you normally use a saw to cut the spine in half lengthwise. Mary started the job but the dead animal was floppy and hard to work with, so I volunteered to finish it with the sword. Without a stroke of any kind, just letting the weight of the blade fall off my shoulder, the steel went through about 18 inches of bone.

Hope that wasn't too gruesome for you. Here's my point; just because something makes perfect sense doesn't mean it is true.

Reason is weak. Most people don't recognize the sheer chaos of survival fighting or the effects that the stress hormones dumped into your bloodstream will have. Seeing a need for training in this area, instructors have a tendency to look at an area they are familiar with and extrapolate it to violence. Many take competition experience or other people's research and try to figure out what "should" work.

Things that should work don't all the time. I've been completely unfazed by a crowbar slamming into the back of my head and been left dizzy and puking for three days from a light slap...also to the back of the head. I couldn't have reasoned that out.

Reason has given rise to a number of martial arts styles, or perhaps fantasy masquerading as reason. There are two ways reason can be applied to any particular aspect of the matrix, such as self-defense. Most people and organizations plan from a "Resources Forward" model. Basically, they look at what they have and figure out what they can do with it. The equivalent in martial arts would be to say, "We're really good at kicking and can punch a little, how do we use that in an ambush?"

"Goals Backwards" looks at the problem and then creates the resources. "What do I need to do, and what do I need to get to accomplish that?" There's no real martial arts equivalent of this thought process. The self-defense equivalent is to ask, "What does a real attack look like, and what do I need to have a chance?" Look at what you need, not what you have. Then you gather what you need instead of trying to stretch resources where they were never meant to go.

In theory, there is no difference between theory and reality.

In reality, there is.

Reason, by itself, is only theory.

Tradition. Often we don't respect the environment that spawned the old combat arts. There is, in my opinion, a persistent myth that we live in the most dangerous and lethal era in human history. Surely our weapons and delivery systems are more powerful, but our perception of the value of life has far outstripped our destructive abilities. For generations raised like I was on the myth of the destructive, wanton Killer Man, this will be a hard sell.

For 2002, the Bureau of Justice statistics put the murder rate at six per 100,000, the lowest rate seen in at least thirty years. Overall violent crime was 25.9 incidents per 1,000. This has shown a steady drop since 1996 (as far back as I was willing to go with some slow-loading tables on their Web site).

I don't know whether those numbers seem low or high to you.

In early 1945, the Battle of Iwo Jima lasted 35 days and resulted in 26,000 dead, combining both sides. The combatants used artillery, bombs, naval guns, and the most sophisticated personal weapons available at the time: rifles, machineguns, flamethrowers, and grenades.

In 1600, the Battle of Sekigahara resulted in about 40,000 dead in six hours. The battle was fought with horses and the most sophisticated personal weapons of the day: swords, spears, bows, and muskets.

It is estimated that the total civilian and military deaths of World War II would be around 50 million people. This was a war where the major industrial nations of the earth fought a war of attrition to the bitter end, a war where nuclear weapons were developed and used.

It is also estimated that using bow and spear and sword, the Mongols conquered Northern China between 1210 and 1240 at the cost of 40 million lives...but they also conquered Russia and the Middle East, another 10 million (perhaps a million in the sack of Baghdad alone) and another five million conquering Southern China from 1250-1280.

Do we really believe that the serial killer is a modern phenomenon? Modern serial killers don't approach the body counts of Elizabeth Bathory who may have killed and bathed in the blood of 600 young women or Gilles de Rais who was eventually executed for the torture, rape, and murder of 200 (more or less) young boys.

What is different today? A countess could not hide behind her nobility and it is difficult and rare to say that peasants don't "count." We have a computer network that helps us know if a murder is part of a larger pattern. We have a media that reports what happens. At the turn of the last century, if someone were killed in your town, no one outside of your county and the relatives would even know—unless it made excellent news, like the Lindbergh baby or the Lizzy Borden ax murders.

We also have the police. The idea was a new concept in the 18th century. The U.S. Marshals Service was founded in 1789. Scotland Yard was founded in 1829. Think about the implications: If you were killed, unless your friends or family sought vengeance, there would be no investigation, no search for justice. You would be forgotten. The killer would move on. Many of these killers lived and worked in bands, sometimes gangs, but sometimes agents of authority. The press gangs beat and kidnapped citizens to "recruit" for the British Navy. The soldiers of the Hundred Years War, the Thirty Years War, and much of the Napoleonic era roamed the countryside supplying themselves, which means robbing, raping, and killing for anything that they wanted or needed. The largely unarmed citizenry had no recourse to any higher authority.

This is the environment and the context in which the older martial arts arose. It was an answer to a primal understanding of violence, something we often miss without the experience to understand and evaluate it.

Anything that is taught becomes tradition. Even a tradition of questioning traditions. Students have a right to know which of their lessons are based on experience and which on reason. Do you even know if the techniques you learn and teach have actually been used? If a martial arts style goes through several generations of teachers without combat experience, will the guesses of the many teachers come to wash away the hard-won experience of the few? Will the rhinoceros become the unicorn?

Entertainment and recreation. Too many people, students of martial arts, concerned citizens, self-defense "experts," and rookie officers learned most of what they think they know from television, movies, or sports events. The purpose of all of these venues is to entertain, not to educate. What they show has been modified to look more interesting. The long, complicated fight scenes of a Hong Kong Kung Fu flick are just as unrealistic as the wire work and flying. In a lethal fight, one party has the advantage or gets it as early as possible and presses it to the quick, brutal end. It's fast. There is very little drama.

Rookie officers come to the academy believing that the right way to make a fast entry is with their weapons next to their heads, pointing at the sky. A technique that only existed so that a cameraman could get the star's face and a gun in the same picture has become something that people who know better try to do. In real life, it is a matter of an instant for a bad guy to grab the barrel and shove it under the officer's chin. A messy death.

Each piece of a well-choreographed movie fight scene is designed to entertain you. The distancing lets the techniques show to best effect. The timing is designed for drama, rhythm, and pacing, not for finishing things. The choice of technique showcases the actor's flexibility.

In combat sports, three major factors make it difficult to extrapolate from the ring to uncontrolled violence. The most critical and hardest to train for is surprise. You know if you have a tournament next Saturday. You know if your club practices free sparring on Monday and Wednesday nights. You do not know when, if ever, you will be attacked. You cannot warm up for it or stretch or eat right or get enough sleep. The second factor is similar—you know what is likely to happen in a combat sport. You know how many opponents you will face and what size they are and whether they will be armed. You know what the footing and lighting will be like. Rules and safety considerations are the third factor. Some rules are instituted for safety. Most grappling styles don't allow fingerlocks or strikes to the brainstem.

Other rules are based on increasing the entertainment value of the art as a spectator sport. Cops pin face down. The samurai used to pin face down and finish things off with a knife in the back of the neck, but wrestling and Judo pin face up because it makes for a better fight if your opponent can use all of his or her weapons.

section 2.4: strategy training

Goals dictate strategy.
Strategy dictates tactics.
Tactics dictate techniques.

Goals differ in different situations. Real violence is a very broad subject and no two encounters are the same. What is a "win" in one situation may not be in the next. The *goal* is how you define the win in that particular encounter. Sometimes it will reflect your martial arts training: An incapacitating blow may be what you need. But sometimes the goal is to break away or create enough space to access a weapon or just get enough air to scream for help. If the goal changes, so does everything else. If you have only trained for one goal, (e.g., the submission), you will be hampered when the goal is different.

If you teach martial arts, start putting your students in situations where the goal is non-standard, such as escaping from a small room or car, drawing a weapon from one of several opponents' belts, or getting to a dummy phone and punching in 911. One of the simplest drills is "Breakthrough" where the student must, as fast as possible, get through a door blocked by two opponents. Fighting each or both of them takes too long.

The goal is what needs to happen; parameters are what need to NOT happen, what you can't do. For me, Departmental Policy and Procedure sets the limits most of the time. But it may also include not leaving someone behind, not losing a weapon from your belt, or any number of limitations. A parameter too few self-defense instructors address is "not getting sued."

Goals and parameters combine to dictate strategy. Strategy is the general plan for accomplishing the goal. Fight, run, and hide are the three classic survival strategies. In the martial arts "Do Damage" is the core strategy of Karate, "Disrupt Balance" is the strategy of Judo.

Individuals and even animals have their own strategies. A wolf pack's goal is meat; the parameter is not getting too injured to survive acquiring the meat. So they choose the weakest animal in the herd, the one least likely to kick effectively. They try to find the weak one when it is isolated from the others and then they try to make it panic and run it to exhaustion, nipping their victim as it tires to weaken it further. Some people do this, too.

Some animals, and some people, wait in ambush. Some technical fighters wait for their opponent to make a mistake that can be exploited. Some sucker-punchers try to distract their victim's attention before they strike. The goal of a quick victory and the parameters of minimal casualties (and the real lack of a parameter in cost and material) result in the military strategy of "Shock and Awe."

Strategy and environment dictate tactics. Tactics are the "how" of implementing strategy. Environment here is used in a very broad sense. Availability of weapons, targets, escape routes, as well as lighting, footing, and space are all elements of the environment that will affect your choice of tactics, as does the information you have and available time.

A SWAT team in a hostage situation will have a general strategy—set up a perimeter, gather intelligence, hope negotiations go well, and be prepared to make an entry if the hostage takers start killing the hostages. They will choose tactics, based on the situation, whether to attempt a stealth entry, a dynamic entry (fast), or an explosive entry (literally using explosives to blow their way in). In addition, they will have set up a hasty plan, a rudimentary set of tactics for entering and saving hostages if the criminals start killing. While one team stands by to implement the hasty plan (limited time, limited information), other elements are working on a better plan, using the time available and any information they can develop.

Tactics and the "totality of circumstances" dictate the specific technique you will use. Totality of circumstances (ToC) is the law enforcement term for all of the infinite details of the moment that influence a decision. Whether you will use a punch or a kick, for example, or a jab versus a cross.

Some examples:

Goal: Stop bad guy (BG) from hurting me
Parameters: None
Strategy: Fight
Environment: Sticks available
Tactic: Hit him with a stick many times
ToC: BG's hands are low
Technique: Snap to the exposed temple

Goal: Stop BG from hurting me
Parameters: Afraid of getting sued
Strategy: Get away
Environment: Exit available
Tactic: Run
ToC: Exit on other side of BG
Technique: Fake left, run right, sprint.

Goal: Prevent two teenagers from attacking
Parameters: Limited time
Strategy: Get help/discourage them
Environment: Cell phone/no bystanders
Tactic: Call for help
ToC: They can hear you and seem uncertain
Technique: Dial 911 and loudly ask for police assistance

Goal: Not be killed by two hostage takers
Parameters: None
Strategy: Run at first opportunity
Environment: Nine hostages, large building
Tactic: Watch for distraction and go
ToC: Threats arguing between themselves
Technique: Sprint when the argument gets heated

If your goals or parameters change, so does everything else. Different situations require different ways of moving, thinking, and acting. Everything changes. Striving for perfection of a single goal, the hallmark of *dojo* training, is far too narrow for real life.

section 2.5: goals in training

In the Reception Line Drill, one student is told that he has been elected Governor and is attending a formal ball held in his honor. The party will start with a reception line where the Governor shakes hands and greets each of the attendees. It is a very important ball and can't be cancelled, even though security believes someone will attempt to assassinate the Governor.

The other students line up while the Governor has his back turned. One of the students in line is given a training knife. The Governor then turns and the line moves past him, shaking his hand, hugging, starting small-talk conversations. This continues until the assassin strikes.

The attack may come while the Governor is shaking hands, after the assassin has passed, or when the line is over and everyone is milling around. There may be no attack at all, especially if the student playing the Governor can't act natural, but seems paranoid and jerky.

I have seen some excellent martial arts when I use this drills at seminars, but I've seen terrible self-defense. After everyone has been through, the chewing-out lecture is almost rote:

"It's not easy to be friendly and flip the switch, is it? There was some good technique; good job.

"There was some bad thinking, though. Did anyone think to yell, 'He's got a knife!'? Or yell for help or tell someone to call the police? Did anybody try to run? There's a damn door right there. This is a *dojo,* for crissakes—there are mirrors everywhere. Did anyone use the mirrors to see who had the knife? Or take a weapon off the wall?

"Each and every one of you handled this like martial artists at a demonstration. Not one of you acted like someone who had to stay alive."

A quick and dirty guide to not being successfully sued:

The legal essence of self-defense is that you are required to use "the minimum level of force" which you "reasonably believe" is necessary to safely resolve the situation.

Minimum level of force: This will tie in to other things in the statement, but if you can solve it with a push, don't use a brick. If you can solve it with a punch, don't use a club; if you can solve it with a club, don't use a knife. Knives and guns, in many places, are interchangeable. Both are considered deadly force. Some manufacturers make knives with brass knuckles attached or designed so that they can be used, opened or closed, as impact weapons or to grind pressure points. Be aware that in many, if not most jurisdictions, even if you do not use it and have no attention of using it as a lethal weapon, it is still legally considered a lethal weapon. In other words, if you use the handle of your knife to poke a pressure point, the legally operative concept is that you have used a knife. No matter how you use it, you must be able to justify deadly force.

The minimum level of force will change in the course of an encounter, sometimes every second. If the threat runs or goes unconscious, stop. You're done. He no longer presents an immediate threat.

Reasonably believe, simply means, would whatever you did be outside the box for another citizen with similar experience and training? If you punch a child who won't stop crying, you're outside the box. It doesn't have to be the same exact technique that each member of the jury would have done, but it has to be within the ballpark.

Reasonably believe applies to and ties together "minimum level" and "necessary."

Necessary: Do you have to do this? Is it your problem? Can you leave? Should you leave? If someone is trashing your store, it is your problem and you can justify acting...if you have to. If the cops will get there in time, you will be expected to at least make the effort to get the professionals involved. Some states have a "duty to retreat" clause written into their self-defense laws that require you to exhaust all available options to get out before you fight back. Usually, it's a good idea any-

---

A quick and dirty guide... *(continued)*

way...however, if someone else may be victimized, you might not be required to leave.

To safely resolve: It is not a contest, not a game, and you are under no requirements to play fair or take chances. If you think you might be able to handle it in a wrestling match but you are sure you can handle it with your umbrella, use the umbrella. This is often a confusing point for civilians watching news telecasts on police issues. The officer is required to handle situations, not at the level in which he will probably prevail, but at the level where he won't get hurt. An injured officer is a drain on resources, possibly another body to be rescued, and certainly not an asset to anyone.

The situation: In general, defense of yourself or a third person from immi-nent harm is legally good self-defense. From that point on, you have to look at state laws. As mentioned before, some have a "duty to retreat." Some have a "castle law" where the homeowner has unfettered rights to self-defense against someone who feloniously breaks into the home. Defense of property also varies from state to state and some jurisdictions have other regulations that restrict permissible self-defense, such as ordinances banning firearms.

Lastly, in order to use force, the person you are using it on must be an immediate threat. In order to be an immediate threat, the threat (my handy law enforcement euphemism for Bad Guy, you'll see it a lot in this book) must exhibit and you must be able to clearly articulate three things:

Intent: You must be able to clearly explain how you knew he was going to hurt you, hurt someone else, kill you, kill someone else, destroy or steal property...whatever the situation you need to resolve. Did he tell you? "I'm gonna kick your fuckin' ass!" That goes in the report. Did he show you? Balling up his fist and moving towards you? Raising a club and charging? Reaching under his jacket where you suspected he had a gun? (Be careful, because you will also have to clearly explain why you thought he had a gun.)

Means: Whatever you feel he was going to do, whatever the situation you had to resolve, you have to be able to articulate that he was able to do

---

A quick and dirty guide... *(continued)*

it. If someone says he's going to shoot you and he has no gun, he has no means. If someone says he's going to beat you up and he's paralyzed from the neck down, he has no means.

Opportunity: If the threat can't reach you, you can't argue that he was an immediate threat. We get "cell warriors" all the time. Locked behind a steel door, they yell threats and challenges. If you open the door, they curl into a little ball and say, "I wasn't talking to you, Sarge." Whatever. However, by opening the door I give them opportunity and if one of these scenarios went bad, it would be my responsibility.

Be aware that in any classroom or *dojo* setting, there is a gap between the perceived goal and the real goal. The perceived goal is what you *think* you are teaching. It may be anything from mastering a technique to learning knife defense. The real goal, the goal the student strives for never changes: Make the instructor happy. If you give the student a self-defense exercise, they will try to do what they think you want them to do, even if it is not the most efficient way to survive.

This is why when you teach scenarios, the students will not go "outside the box" without specific permission. They won't scream or yell at another student to dial 911, or run away or grab a weapon off the wall—all things they should really do if attacked—because deep down the goal is to give the instructor what the students think the instructor wants.

section 2.6: thinking in the moment

Strategy and tactics, assumptions and epistemology are all critical to thinking about violence and preparing for violence. In the moment of sudden attack, however, your brain will change. The way you think will change. The section on the "Chemical Cocktail" (*See* Section 3.3) will cover some of those chemical changes. Right here, we will discuss the mechanics of decision making in a violent encounter.

The OODA loop, described by U.S. Air Force Colonel John Boyd, has become the standard nomenclature for combative decision-making. In essence, each person must: *Observe* what is happening; *Orient* to the observations (interpret the sensory input); *Decide* what to do about it; and *Act*.

This isn't new—I remember one martial arts instructor from long ago who had the "Four Ps": Perceive, Present, Plan, Perform. My *sensei* taught it as the elements of speed—perceptual speed, interpretation by experience, the decision tree, and then neuromuscular speed. The basic idea isn't new or even fresh, but OODA has become standard.

Clarifying example:
O: You see a fist suddenly growing larger. (observe)
O: Hey, that must mean it is getting closer! I'm being punched! (orient)
D: What should I do about it? Block or duck? Duck! (decide)
A: Duck! (act)

I was taught these as the elements of speed with the caution that reactive moves, such as blocking, rarely work because the bad guy is on step four when his action triggers your step one. His "act" is the first thing you "observe."

Time is most critically lost in the two middle steps. In the orientation step, inexperienced people try to gather too much or too little information. In combat or self-defense, the usual problem is to try to get too much information. I need to know where his good targets and my available weapons are. That is all. Martial artists tend to also want to know how he reacted to their last attack and what he is likely to do next. That's chess thinking, not brawl thinking—predicting what the threat will do in four moves is useless if the intervening three moves are stabs. The most fatal decision in an ambush is the "why" question—"Why are they doing this?" "What does this mean?" You won't get an answer and if you did get an answer, it wouldn't help you. But many, many victims freeze right here, with the "why."

Decide is the second time waster. There's a thing called Hick's Law, which states that the more options you have, the longer it takes to choose one. Makes sense. I call this the Brown Belt Syndrome. It's what happens when you have too many cool ways to win and you get your ass kicked while you are weighing your options. The way to grow past this is something I call "meta-strategy." Again, this is something I've back-engineered from the people that consistently make it work, not something I'm reasoning out.

The people I know who consistently do well in ambushes or have often beaten the maxim that action is faster than reaction have one thing in common. They have a group of techniques that form the core of their strategy that they DO NOT SEE AS SEPARATE TECHNIQUES. Mac has hundreds of disarms and counterattacks, but when he is surprised he "de-fangs the snake." He can and will do it in a hundred different ways, but in his mind it's just one thing. James "does damage." Again, hundreds of techniques that are all one thing in his brain. I "take the center."

Operant conditioning (*See* Section 5.4) is critical in self-defense because it is possible, in certain situations, including surprise attacks, to cut out the middle two steps and develop an automatic, reflex-level response.

Two or more people in conflict have their OODA loops activated and they feed off each other. My actions are your observations. When what you observe changes, you must reorient. If I can conclude my loop faster, I not only act faster and get more damage in, but I also throw you off your loop. If you start to swing and I hit you in the face, most people will stop their swing to reorient.

The closer the events reflect previous experience, the less time it takes to orient. If the event is completely new, such as a *judoka* experiencing his first leg lock, it is effectively invisible—there is nothing in the past to orient to (which explains the effectiveness of Judo in 1888, Jujutsu in America in the 1920s, Karate in the '50s, and Brazilian Jujitsu in the '90s). This is also the purpose of cognitive interrupts or context shifting: doing something, such as blowing a kiss or drooling that doesn't compute as a fight. In short, you can attack the OODA loop as well as attacking the body.

Exploiting the OODA loop:

(1) People lock up on novel observations. If you observe something and can't tell what it is (a giant carnivorous tomato with

tentacles or someone clearing his throat, preparing to spit to open a combat), you can't orient to it, so you can't decide or act. Someone commented that people are never brave (read decisive) in conditions of uncertainty. One of the goals of training must be to expose yourself to the widest variety of situations possible to prevent this.

(2) You must be able to act with partial information. You will never have all the answers or know exactly what is going on. People who wait for too much information before acting get hurt. The speed of your OODA loop depends on your comfort level of information.

(3) The person with a plan or an internal map of what is supposed to happen will have a hard time orienting if the plan isn't followed. The attacker who has chosen a small female may have laid a detailed plan: He will grab her by the hair and when she screams, he will slap her; and if she continues to scream, he will... If the actual events go more like "he grabs her hair and his nose explodes in blood and pain," he will have a momentary freeze as he orients to the unexpected events.

(4) Each action on your part is a new observation. The power in a barrage attack or a fast entry in a tactical situation is because the constant action constantly resets the opponent's OODA loop. Observe: "His fist is getting big." Orient: "He's hitting..." Observe: "His other fist is getting big." Orient: "It's a combo!" Observe: "My knee just collapsed." Orient: "He's kicking, too!" The constant attack keeps the opponent bouncing between the first two steps, never deciding or acting.

(5) (And this is wicked cool!) This can be defeated by a self-referencing stimulus. Barrages haven't worked on me. Chain punches haven't worked on me. The reason is that when my senses get overwhelmed, I shut down the source of the information. To put it in OODA terms, if I feel myself caught in the OO bounce or sense it about to happen, I attack. The OO bounce has become an observation in and of itself with a simple one-choice orient ("I'm frozen") followed by a simple decision: "Hit the bastard!" and a simple action—*POW!*

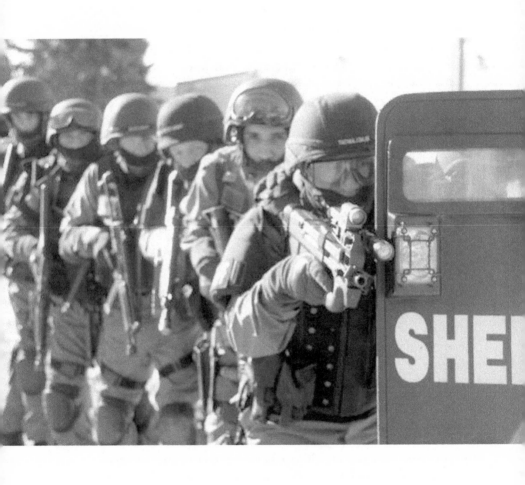

CHAPTER 3: VIOLENCE

section 3.1: types of violence

Most humans fight for status or territory like other animals. Most conflict is about "face" or "respect," not about necessity. The need to establish a place in the hierarchy of humans is a very powerful drive, one that influences many humans for much of their lives. The fear of being challenged on this basis is also overwhelming and is expressed in many ways. Most people have a fear of talking in public. Many people find it difficult to ask an attractive stranger for a date without alcohol.

No one can argue that this fear and reluctance are based on a probability of injury. All that the person stands to lose is self-image, status. Fear of losing this imaginary thing drives a huge amount of violence from gang shootings to inmate assaults to spouse abuse.

That is the first distinction: to understand the difference between violence for status and image versus violence for resources.

Here's a concept we will revisit again and again in this book: You are not you. Who you think you are, the story you tell yourself every day, is an illusion. Humans are animals with very real animal needs and senses plugged in to a living, primal animal world. At the same time, people are bundles of history and interaction and decision and compromise. Somewhere in the mist, between your animal self and your decisions, you tell a story to yourself.

Are you the brave and independent woman standing up for herself in the world of men? The terrifying thing about rape isn't the physical damage—that usually heals. It's the destruction of this image.

Are you a generally good guy, willing to stand up for what's right? That's why your mouth goes dry and your stomach knots up when someone flips you off in traffic or yells a threat—because when the rubber hits the road, you may not be who you think you are. You may lose or you might even run. Or crawl. Or beg.

SWAT stack
Courtesy Antonio B. Urena

This story you tell yourself is something you have built up since birth. In a very real sense, it is your life's work. The damage to the story can have longer-term effects than damage to the body. The risk to the story, to your self-image, status, and ego can generate far more fear than mere physical risk.

It doesn't make any sense, but people are weird that way.

Patterns of Violence

The Monkey Dance. Remember the saying: "When two tigers fight, one is killed and one is maimed"? That's a lie. How often have you watched a nature special on TV and seen two grizzlies growling and biting, shoving and clawing? When it's over, one walks away relatively unscathed and the other keeps the territory.

Bighorn sheep rams square off and charge head to head, slamming blocks of horn over bone together until one wanders off and the other keeps the herd of females. If the loser circled around, came back and slammed the winner in the ribs, he would kill him…but they don't do that. This kind of conflict is a ritual with genetically built-in safety measures.

Humans are apes and we have our own built-in ritual combat to establish social dominance or defend territory. It is nearly always non-lethal. I call it the Monkey Dance.

The Monkey Dance is a ritual, with specific steps. The dance, I believe, is innate. The steps may be cultural. In my culture:

Eye contact, hard stare.

Verbal challenge, (e.g. "What you lookin' at?").

Close the distance. Sometimes chest bumping.

Finger poke or two-handed push to the chest.

Dominant hand roundhouse punch. A very experienced friend has told me that even left handers tend to throw a right-hand punch, which would be a good argument for genetic predetermination, but I never thought to ask if anyone was left handed after an incident.

Most martial arts (and most adolescent combat fantasies) are based on this model. It is much easier to prevail in a scenario that is already genetically designed to be nonlethal.

The listed step shows only one side of the dance. At each step, the other monkey answers. Think about the number of times you have seen this pattern or participated in it:

"What you lookin' at?"

"None of your business. Fuck you."

"Oh yeah?" Closes, chests almost touching, "What you got to say now, motherfucker?"

"Get up outta my face or deal."

"Yeah?" Chest shove.

"Don't put your hands on me!"

Swing.

Once you feed into this contest, you are no longer in control. It is the product of millennia of evolution. I want to make this perfectly clear: No matter how much I refer to the Monkey Dance as a dominance game, you do not play it. It plays you.

Because it is all about dominance, you can usually circumvent the dance with submissive body language, such as lowering your eyes and apologizing. This has a personal cost, however. For most men, backing down from a status conflict is very difficult and does psychological damage.

To understand, think about where this ritual came from. Loose bands of people, living on the edge of subsistence, dependent on each other, and yet competing for scarce resources. In many cases, like many species, only the very high status males bred. You were only born because a long string of your ancestors successfully played this game. That's a lot of conditioning. In this imaginary band, the alpha males bred. Another loose category struggled for alpha status, and the lowest of the low DIDN'T struggle for it. They had accepted, probably out of fear, a status so low as to be beneath notice.

A friend of mine is an author. He's a good man, retired from good service to the community, a wise friend with a good family. He doesn't remember the fights that he won and lost growing up, but he does remember the one fight he backed down from. In third grade, he was challenged by a bully and ran. Nearly seventy years later, it still haunts him. You will find this scarring in many people, if you look. They did not act the way the person in their private story was supposed to.

The key to avoiding the damage is to purposely avoid the dance. If you meekly lower your eyes and apologize out of fear, you will feel terrible about it. If you do it consciously, as a ploy, it is far less damaging but de-escalates the situation pretty reliably.

Another method of de-escalation requires confidence. Have you watched a big dog ignoring a pack of puppies that are playing at their little dominance games? The dog understands instinctively that he can only participate in the dominance game if he feels one of the pups is a legitimate challenge to his authority. He actually lowers his status immeasurably by participating.

In the Big Dog tactic, you maintain extremely relaxed body language and treat the verbal challenges as serious, thoughtful questions.

"What you lookin' at?"

I put my hands behind my head and put my feet up on the desk. "Just zoning for a minute. Worked a double yesterday. How you doin'?"

Acting bored and thoughtful can be very powerful. By not questioning your own status, it makes it harder for someone to challenge you for it. There is more, however. Boredom itself is one of the big indicators of confidence and even status. Whether it is in a boardroom, a job interview, a duel, or a football game, nervousness is the sign of the underdog, the probable loser. The opposite of nervousness can go beyond calm into bored. Powerful.

There are two related concepts that can manifest in apparent boredom: the Japanese concept of *zanshin* and the American concept of "cool."

In biology and animal psychology I was taught that animals could tell, often by smell and almost immediately, if a stranger of the same species were higher or lower in status. If two hierarchies of rats are thrown together, the new hierarchy is forged by animals of similar levels fighting. The beta male doesn't attack the alpha male.

Humans have this ability. They can often sense danger, authority, or weakness in another human. More importantly, certain people can project an aura of confidence or competence that others read as a clear signal NOT to Monkey Dance.

The Japanese concept for the ability to project this aura is *zanshin*. The word gets translated many ways: as "awareness," "remaining mind," or "indomitable will." It is always tied to BOTH awareness and experience. In my personal belief, the *bushi* (Japanese warriors) recognized that this aura is cultivated by a combination of awareness and insight into experience.

Though some can put on a good show for a while, there is a huge difference in feel and information between the people who have put their lives on the line and the ones who have only read or day-dreamed about it. A self-defense expert who has read DeBecker and Christensen and MacYoung and Strong and Blauer will be able to get good information to their students—in a very real sense, they will know the words, but not the music.

Experience is only a part of *zanshin*. If you don't pay attention to the experience, it might as well not have happened. A person can go to hell and back, but if he spent the trip covering his eyes and chanting, "This isn't happening. This isn't happening," he will not develop *zanshin*. If you live in denial, hiding from the experience and its effects, you will not develop *zanshin*.

You must have the experience. You must make the experience part of you by examining it and seeking to understand it—by mining the experience for its lessons.

The concept of *zanshin* is also tied to awareness: In the situations where experience accumulates, you don't do well unless you are alert. I tell people that being a jail guard is a very safe, very easy job for smart people who pay attention...and a dangerous, difficult job for stupid people who don't pay attention. Heightened awareness is also rewarded and you will find that veterans of long-term military combat (for example) do not use their eyes, ears, noses, or skin the way that civilians do. For example, some people associate the "1,000-yard stare" with shell shock. It's actually a way to use the eyes to detect movement very efficiently and increase peripheral vision.

Veterans don't process the sensory information in the same way as civilians, either—they often ignore the social context. It is very rare for a combat veteran to decide not to duck out of fear of "looking silly."

There is a correlation to *zanshin* in our culture: cool. A person can be cool under fire or cool headed or just a cool dude. In all cases, it is a projected aura of competence.

My first professional experience in this field was working as a bouncer in a casino. We were escorting a foul-mouthed drunk out and he turned and swung. I ducked and he connected solidly with my partner. Two hot young martial artists versus a drunk and it turned into a wrestling match under the roulette table. Our boss came down from his coffee break. Jim was old—he'd retired from the military as an MP and then retired from a police force. He'd come to work as a shift supervisor in the casino simply because he couldn't imagine not working.

He came down the stairs with a cigarette dangling from his lip, a full cup of coffee in his hand, and casually walked over and knelt on the drunk's neck. The drunk went limp. Jim took a sip of his coffee and said, "You boys think you got this from here?" Then he went back upstairs to finish his pie. He didn't spill his coffee. Jim was cool. Jim had *zanshin*.

There are other demeanors that remove you from the status contest. The Monkey Dance is based on gaining status and many who play it want a quick back-down with minimal risk. Very few people challenge children, for instance. There is no status to gain. No one plays the Monkey Dance with a crazy person—there is little chance for status, no guarantee of a quick back-down, and crazy people don't always follow the steps.

If it's appropriate, circumvent the Monkey Dance by jumping steps. If the threat is at any level below contact and you attack, you will cause him to freeze. The dance is a biological game and it takes a small amount of time to adjust when someone cheats. Many people will consider this kind of preemptive strike unjustifiable. Just be sure that you can articulate Intent, Means, and Opportunity. This preemptive movement is the perfect time and psychological set-up that allows an experienced officer to handle a threat with low level techniques such as joint locks.

Rarely can anyone make a joint lock work against a strike outside the conditions of a *dojo* with people trained to strike in a certain and ineffective way. If the officer waited for the threat to strike, the officer might be forced to strike or even use a weapon—a high risk of injury solution. By jumping steps, the officer is able to resolve the situation at a lower level, with less risk of injury to everyone.

The Monkey Dance described here is a male phenomenon. It is very rare in nature for the female of the species to dispute for status and territory. Females are less genetically expendable than men and the loss, no matter how small in intraspecies competition, would damage the evolutionary chances of the species or tribe.

Do the math. Imagine two tribes, each with twenty people. Each tribe has ten men and ten women. Tribe X uses its men to do the fighting; Tribe Z uses its women. The two tribes go to war. It's a stalemate, but each tribe loses three warriors. The next year, tribe X has seven warrior fathers, ten stay-at-home moms, and ten babies. Tribe Z has seven warrior moms, ten stay-at-home dads, and only seven babies. Tribe population is now 27 to 24. If they lose five warriors the next year, Tribe X will still have ten babies; Tribe Z will have only two. Women are too valuable genetically to risk in dominance games in a marginal society.

So women haven't been bred to deal with this kind of conflict.

This has powerful effects that must be addressed in intergender conflicts.

First, remember that the Monkey Dance is biologically designed to be nonlethal. Damage when it occurs is usually cosmetic. Fatalities, when they do occur, are nearly always due to falling and hitting the head. Just as women do not have the ritual of dominance-based violence, they also lack the built-in safety. In other words, if you are dealing with a female threat, she will be seeking to do damage, not to show who is boss. In my experience, women gouge for eyes, bite, and try to cut the face with their fingernails far more often than men.

Second, if you are a woman dealing with a male threat, he can still Monkey Dance at you and perceive you to be challenging him. A significant percentage of the males who prey on women are seeking to safely establish dominance over somebody. In that case, when a woman fights back the man will react very violently. In his mind, a victim specially chosen to be weak enough to guarantee his validation as a dominator has seen him as weak enough to challenge. A man fighting another man for dominance will try to beat him, but a man who thinks that he is fighting a woman for dominance will be seeking to punish her. Punishment is much worse.

Third, there are specific reactions to violence that most women have absorbed at a very young age that profoundly affect their ability to defend themselves. You see this in victims who flirt with or compliment their attacker: "You're so handsome you don't need to rape." And you see it in women who struggle instead of fight. Women are used to handling men in certain ways, with certain subconscious rules—social ways, not physical ones. These systems are very effective within society and not effective at all when civilization is no longer a factor, such as in a violent assault or rape.

On a deep level, most women feel at a gut level that if they fight a man he will escalate the situation to a savage beating, punishment for her challenge to his "manhood." They feel this way because it is true. This is a hard thing to write. Years ago, before I learned to just listen, a friend told me her story. It had been several days and most of the swelling had gone down. She told me about the rape and the beating. I asked her if she had fought. Not my business and decades of experience later I would have just listened, but I was young and believed that there were more right and wrong answers than there are. She shook her head and said, "I was afraid he'd hurt me if I fought."

This fear of escalation is based on unknowns. The attacker has already decided to hurt the victim and largely how much. The feared "greater level of damage" is only in relation to the level of damage, unknown to you, that the threat has already planned.

If he is already planning to torture and kill, the feared escalation is meaningless, but you can't know his plan at the outset. The choice must be yours, made in an instant and on incomplete information. A fear of provoking a beating or torture or death will not help you if the attacker has already decided on a beating or torture or death.

Do not interpret anything I say here to mean "don't fight back." I'm also not going to patronize you with half-truths or platitudes. This is ugly on many levels: the level of the incident and the level of social conditioning to "get along," which can make it so much harder to decide not to be a victim.

This means that if and when a woman chooses to fight, it must be a total effort. In many cases, there is no level of force that will simply discourage a male attacker. He must be incapacitated. This is my advice and I think this mindset is critical, but the actual statistics are less grim—many assailants do run away and do not escalate when they encounter unexpected resistance.

The Group Monkey Dance. I had some criminals in custody for a long time. There were several codefendants involved, but I remember two: one was a skinny, pale kid, crying and begging me to put him in protective custody because he was afraid "the real criminals in here will steal my food." The other was a young lady, intelligent and articulate. If you imagine the heavy girl with glasses from high school, the one who was on the chess team, you'll have a good mental picture.

They were in custody for the savage torture, beating, murder, and burning of a developmentally-disabled woman. Neither of them fit my profile of a predatory killer, and yet they killed.

The Group Monkey Dance (GMD) is another dominance game. In this ritual, members of a group compete for status and to show their loyalty to the group by showing how vicious they can be to someone perceived as an "outsider." It is purely a contest to prove who is more a part of the group by who can do the most violence to the outsider.

To someone who has never seen, investigated, or been involved in the GMD, it is hard to describe. It is hard to explain how completely inconsequential the victim is. Once the dance starts, the victim is literally a non-person. Any action—pleading, fighting, passivity—will be interpreted by the group as proof of "otherness" and further justification to escalate.

Some of the most brutal assaults and murders have been the result of a GMD. When you think of mobs erupting into violence or the unbelievable brutality and destruction of a prison riot or a Central Park "wilding," you are thinking of the GMD. When you see soldiers mutilated and their bodies dragged through villages, you are witnessing a version of the GMD. Sometimes even death of the outsider doesn't stop the dance.

The psychology behind this is probably what allowed normal citizens to become death camp guards in WWII. Some people—leaders of violent terrorist or political movements and criminal bosses—use this tendency to influence their followers to kill. In every war, both sides have had a slang term for the enemy to depersonalize them and make them easier to kill, an attempt to emphasize the "otherness."

Normal people, even good people, can get caught up in the dynamic. In law enforcement, we call it a "feeding frenzy." Usually rookie officers, seeing a Use of Force and still eager to prove themselves, will jump in, which is fine. Usually, the more officers involved, the less risk of injury. However, if one officer escalates the Use of Force to a higher level than is justified, others may follow suit. If one continues after the threat is restrained, others may follow suit.*

The receiving end of the GMD is an ugly, ugly situation. Early in the encounter you may be able to personalize yourself, share information in such a way that most of the members can't see you as an "other." But that will only work in incidents with long preludes, such as some hostage scenarios. Two nonphysical de-escalations have worked for me. In one, I pretended to be crazy, faking a "thorazine twitch" and holding an animated conversation with Jesus and Elvis. In the other (this is subtle), I acted like a tough guy while making it obvious that I was much younger and smaller than they were. The tactic allowed them to laugh at me without having to prove anything. Call it the "little puppy" corollary to the Big Dog technique.

Some have survived by running and hiding, a few by playing dead, others by a counterattack of such awe-inspiring violence that

---

*Calm, in this type of incident, is just as contagious as viciousness. It will be especially powerful coming from the highest rank member of the group (not always rank as in job title, so much as rank in the informal hierarchy). A friend had one of his first uses of force with a lieutenant and me. He later said, "I was getting pretty jacked up and then I looked at the LT and she was dead calm and I looked at you and you looked bored so I figured there wasn't anything to get excited about." One of my primary criteria for CERT recruits is a reputation for not getting excited in a fight. I don't want eager hotshots. I want bored, experienced veterans.

> ## "Multiple officers decrease risk of injury."
>
> I'm going to explain that statement here so that it doesn't interrupt the flow of thought, and because it describes an important principle. If you are a bad guy, huge, and vicious but unarmed, and I am alone, I need to use as much force as I reasonably believe will get me out of there alive. Preferably, I'll get handcuffs on you, too.
>
> The idea of using non-harmful restraint techniques against a really aggressive threat is pretty much fantasy. It's hard to catch a fist in the air, impossible to catch a flurry.
>
> If I am alone with a big, aggressive threat, I will hurt him. I will hit him in the way I believe will most likely keep him from hurting me. That means hard, fast, and targeted. One of us is going to a hospital. My job is to make sure it's not me.
>
> If I have six guys to help me, the principle doesn't change: I need to use as much force as I reasonably believe will get me out of there alive. The difference is that we can assign one guy to each limb, one to control the head, and one to help with anything that gets loose...we can use sheer mass to tire him out and get the cuffs on.
>
> Alone, I can almost guarantee serious injury. With enough help, I can almost guarantee no serious injury.

the group was terrified. A friend and fellow officer (who also happens to be strong, quick, a champion wrestler, and nearly 400 pounds) faced with a mass of inmates starting to riot grabbed the biggest, spun him over his head, and slammed him onto the ground at his feet. "Anyone else? No? Good decision. Go to your bunks."

There is a lower level of GMD. It happens sometimes when "outsiders" are seen to be intruding into an "in-house" dispute. This is the mechanism behind the victim in a spouse abuse case turning on the responding officers, or a pair of young fighters and sometimes the audience turning on a stranger who is trying to break up a fight. This level is rarely as vicious as the GMD—the group merely wants the outsider out. It does not often turn into a brutality contest.

It is still dangerous, very dangerous as many officers who have responded to domestic calls will attest. Not only will the bad guy fight, but sometimes the person you are trying to help as well. But they probably won't drag your body through the street.

Predatory Violence. Violence with a goal beyond domination is not like the Monkey Dance. It more closely mimics the violence between different species.

There is an old tale in many martial arts about a Shaolin monk who went out one morning to meditate and watched a crane fighting a snake. The crane used sweeps of its wings as defense and offense combined with sharp strikes from its beak and kicks. The monk was so impressed with the movement of the crane that he founded the Crane or White Crane system of Kung Fu. The Crane style became the ancestor of many styles in Southern China and Okinawa.

That is a pretty story. It's also utter horseshit.

Cranes don't fight snakes: They kill them. How does a crane do it? It moves very, very slowly and finds the slowest, stupidest, fattest, and most lethargic snake it can and it spears* it through the back.

When a bear wrestles with another bear for dominance, it is nothing like the ambush and charge that the bear uses on an elk. When tigers battle for territory, the loser leaves. The very fact that he is able to leave indicates that the other tiger did not treat him like a water buffalo. The dominance ritual of rattlesnakes can be mistaken for mating unless you are an observant herpetologist and notice that both the snakes involved are male—it's nothing like the way rattlers kill mice.

In predatory violence, the victim is a resource. The attack is a planned, efficient, and safe way for the attacker to get what he wants from that resource. It is not a contest. It is not a fight. It looks and feels nothing like competition at any level.

Generally, human predators use two distinct strategies to approach and disable their human victims. The blitz attack is the sudden, brutal assault from ambush. The threat will get as close as he can without being noticed or triggering a defensive response and then attempt to

---

*I am aware that cranes bite rather than "spear"; it just makes for a better image this way. However, if this story is passed on by word of mouth, faithfully for generations, there will be martial artists in the next century who will believe that cranes spear with their beaks.

overwhelm the victim physically and mentally with a fast, vicious attack.

The second attack strategy uses charm and persuasiveness to get close enough and keep the victim off-guard. It then progresses like a blitz, with an overwhelming onslaught.

[*Generalization alert*: The worst attacks happen this way and these are the situations that it is most critical to prepare for but in the interest of accuracy, I must tell you that the most common attack for a male on female assault was: "1. The victim was approached from the rear/side/front, a threat was made with a weapon, and then the weapon was hidden.

Then the victim's right upper arm was held by the attacker's left hand and the victim was led away." From the excellent article "Condition Black: Assault in Progress" by R. J. Nash.]

Gavin DeBecker, in his book *The Gift of Fear,* has detailed the ploys that predators use to get close to victims. I can't improve on that list and recommend the book. For now, think of one key point: People are not charming, it is not an inherited trait. Charm is something people use, a conscious act to get what they want. There are no charming people, only people who use charm.

The predatory threat has a goal—your money, rape, or to live out a long-held fantasy. His actions are to further that goal at the least risk to himself. He chooses his victim, picking someone who looks weak, distracted, and passive; chooses a time and a place where everything is in the predator's advantage; and strikes suddenly and decisively.

Though the dynamics of the attack are similar, there are two distinct types of predators. All predators see the victim as a resource. For some, the goal is something, tangible or intangible, that they will have after or at the end of the attack. Money. The rape. Status. Drugs.

For a very few, the point of the attack is the attack itself. The torture murder or torture rape follows a different dynamic than the "simple" crime. These are predators who have scripted a fantasy of the crime in their imagination. They are acting out that fantasy. Call them "process predators."

Regular predators are more likely to run in packs than process predators.

Very, very few martial artists have a realistic idea of a predatory attack in their training assumptions.

section 3.2: the four basic truths of violent assault

I investigated an incident between two inmates, an assault. As you read the description, be aware that this is the norm for a solo, un-armed attack. It is not special or unusual in any way.

One was brushing his teeth. The other came up behind him and struck him on the right side of his head. The tooth brusher tried to turn but was pressed into a corner, punched again and again with hard rights until he curled into a fetal ball. Blood splashed (not smeared) onto the wall at shoulder height.

The attacker broke several bones in his hand and did not know it. Not only did he break his own metacarpals in what is called a "boxer's fracture," but he also had one finger deformed, bent, and twisted to the side. Until I pointed it out, he didn't know it. He started complaining of the pain hours after the assault. His hand was broken, but he kept hitting.

I told the attacker that he was lucky—if the other guy had fallen or hit his head on the wall and suffered more serious injury, he could be looking at some heavier charges.

He said, "Nah, I held his head with my other hand so it wouldn't hit the wall. I know how you guys trump up charges and if I'd let him hit the wall, you'd try to get me for attempted murder." In the midst of this ambush, he was thinking.

Most martial artists are completely unprepared for this. Most civilians, who have learned what they know of fighting by watching carefully staged and choreographed movie scenes or skilled competitors in a test of skill and cunning, can't really relate to it. Do you respect the power of a sudden attack and a constant barrage, a "Shock and Awe" of speed and pain that comes on faster than your mind can process? Do you believe that there is a level of pain alone that will stop a committed attacker? Do you believe that a broken nose or the pain of a broken hand is a fight ender? Do you and the politicians and lawyers and judges really realize how rational a sudden assault can be? It's only sudden for the defender. For the attacker, it is planned. Do the politicians who write policy and statute understand that there is a sub-group of human beings who can savagely beat another human being while coolly thinking of their eventual court case?

The four truths: Assaults happen closer, faster, more suddenly, and with more power than most people believe.

Closer. One of the most common and artificial aspects of modern martial arts training is that self-defense drills are practiced at an optimum distance where the attacker must take at least a half step to contact. Real criminals rarely give this luxury of time. They strike when they are sure of hitting, positive that their victim is well within range before initiating the attack.

That half step of extra distance allows many things to work that are hard to pull off in real life. Blocks and evasions rarely work in real encounters. (*See* Section 6.1: Stages of Defense) Even in the *dojo*, if you stand close enough that you can lay your forearm on your partner's shoulder (nearly optimum striking range) and allow him to strike with either hand to targets of his choice, you will not block the strikes in time unless he telegraphs badly. Distance IS time, and blocking takes time.

The attacker always chooses the time and place for the attack, and he chooses a range at which he can surely hit hard and his victim will have the least possible time to react. This means he will be close. Often, the ambush place will be an area that hampers the victim's movements—a toilet stall, between two parked cars or slammed into a wall. Will your favorite move still work without the room to turn or step?

Faster. Because the threat has chosen the time, the place, and the victim, he can attack all-out, with no thought given to defense. The speed of this flurry, the constant rain of blows, can be mind numbing.

When your martial arts students are sparring, use a stopwatch and time how many blows are thrown in a minute. Even in professional boxing, the number is not that impressive. There is a give and take to sparring and subtleties of timing in defense and offense that are integral to making it a game of skill.

Then time them on the heavy bag. Instruct them to hit as fast as they can for ten seconds. Choose a five-second interval early in the drill and count how many blows land. Tips: (1) It is easier to count by sound than sight; (2) don't try to count past twenty; when you get to twenty, hold up one finger and start back at one; (3) if you try to say the numbers, even mentally, you won't be fast enough.

Completely untrained people usually do four hits a second. Eight to ten times a second is reasonable for a decent martial artist. Thirteen to fourteen is the highest I've done.

An assault is conducted like this flurry, not like sparring. A competent martial artist who is used to the more cautious timing of sparring is completely unprepared for this kind of speed. Even the people who strike ten times a second can't block ten times a second.

More Suddenly. An assault is based on the threat's assessment of his chances. If he can't get surprise, he often won't attack. Some experts say that there is always some intuitive warning. Possibly, but if the warning was noted and heeded, the attack would be prevented. When the attack happens, it is always a surprise.

This is one of the hardest aspects of an ambush to train for. The very fact that you know you are training removes the element of surprise. The unexpectedness of an attack can negate nearly any skill. You psych up for training, for competition. You have time to use breathing techniques to adjust your adrenalin balance in class, but an assault happens while you are in your nine to five mind; when your brain is dealing with bills or shopping lists or lost car keys.

More Power. There is a built-in problem with all training. You want to recycle your partners. If you or your students hit as hard as they can every time they hit, you will quickly run out of students.

Truthfully, the average criminal does not hit nearly as hard as a good boxer or *karateka* can hit. They do hit harder than the average boxer (because of gloves) or *karateka* has ever felt.

Being hit is part of the normal environment of an attack. More often than not, the first strike in an ambush lands. So do many others. It can be a sharp and stinging pain, not like the dull ocean roar of a boxing hit or a kind of wincing where part of your face wants to curl over the point of impact. Good martial artists, good ring fighters often freeze for a second because the attack doesn't *feel* like training. If anything feels, sounds, or smells different than you have trained for, your body will be aware that it is a new experience and might freeze. Fighting with a concussion doesn't feel like sparring. (*See* the discussion of "Training and Experience" in Section 3.4).

section 3.3: the chemical cocktail

When you are put under extreme stress, various glands in your body release hormones into the bloodstream that have a profound affect on you physically and mentally. The cocktail analogy is very apt. There are differences in the hormones based on the source and intensity of stress, and the cocktail affects different people in slightly different ways. Think bourbon and sake, happy drunks and mean drunks. Feel the emotional difference between rock climbing and public speaking. Different cocktails.

When this affect hits, your body and mind change. This is one of the hardest things to address in training. The mind you train with will not be the one you have when attacked. This is a key problem. Very often, martial arts are an attempt to come up with a logical, mental answer to a chaotic, visceral problem.

It is also very, very easy for students and teachers to either deny that this affect exists or to pretend that they can train it away. Flat out, breathing control only works to control the affects if you have time to use it. If you have time to take a series of breaths in a specific way to calm yourself down, the time and effort would usually be better spent leaving. Visualization works to give you a plan but doesn't, to my experience, take the edge off the adrenaline. You can believe that if you train hard, you'll be okay. But do not let yourself believe that if you train hard your body won't have natural physiological reactions. Some rely on the concept of *mushin*. I'll write about that in more detail later, but *mushin* is the concept that your body will do what it needs to do with the conscious mind turned off. The state does exist. It is very useful. It comes from dedicated, repetitive training. I can't say it won't be there for you...if you have either experienced a lot of attacks or the particular attack matches your training very, very closely, it might. Don't count on it.

There is a statistic floating around: "At seven yards or less, officers miss 92% of the time." I've heard this statistic from our police academy and in training sessions with the U.S. Marshals. I have no idea where it came from and I haven't been able to find the source. However, NYPD statistics from 1994–2000 show a hit percentage at zero to two yards of 38%. Think about that—a trained officer at contact range to six feet away misses 62% of the time. At the firing range, it would be almost unheard of to miss at six feet.

At three to seven yards, they missed 83% of the time.

There's more going on here than just the chemical cocktail. Just as a hand-to-hand fight is not like sparring, getting an accurate shot in a dark, slick, rainy alley while some tweaker slashes at you with a rusty knife doesn't have a lot in common with firing tight little groups at the range. But the chemical cocktail is part of it. In all likelihood, you've been scared enough to have the shakes, to feel your mouth go dry, and your knees shake. You've wiped the sweat from your palms. Would it be easy to kick with your knees shaking like that? Hold a proper fist with your hand shaking?

Skilled technique degrades under stress. It degrades a lot. If you've ever heard or said, "If it was for real, I would have done better," you've bought into a huge lie. When the stakes are higher, people do much, much worse than when the pressure is low.

For a noncombat example, imagine a college-age young man. He's intelligent, holds witty conversations with his friends and family, and can strike up a conversation with a complete stranger and keep it going. This same young man, when he finally works up the nerve to ask the girl of his dreams on a date, will turn into a babbling idiot. It is a similar mix of hormones with a similar degradation of skills. In most cases, the young man's fighting skills in a real altercation will degrade about as much as his talking skills did in this scenario.

Some of the hormonal affects are physical. Under the stress hormones, peripheral vision is lost and there is physical "tunnel vision." Depth perception is lost or altered, resulting in officers remembering a threat five feet away as down a forty-foot corridor. Auditory exclusion occurs—you may not hear gunfire, or people shouting your name or sirens.

Blood is pooled in the internal organs, drawn away from the limbs. Your legs and arms may feel weak and cold and clumsy. You may not be able to feel your fingers and you will not be able to use "fine motor skills," the precision grips and strikes necessary for some styles such as Aikido.

Complex motor skills, essentially your coordination, will be hampered with a strong enough cocktail. Trapping, combinations, throws—anything that requires hands and feet working together will be gone.

Part is also mental. Perception and memory can be wildly distorted. You may remember nothing, a blur, or incredibly precise details of inconsequential items. Time may seem to slow (tachypsychia). You may freeze and see everything happen but not be able to move...or you may think that you aren't moving when you are, but you are *perceiving* it in slow motion.

Irrelevant thoughts will intrude. This is difficult to describe, but I've been in a fight and suddenly become obsessed with trying to remember what flavor our wedding cake was.

Sometimes the irrelevant thoughts will seem like brilliant ideas or legitimate concerns that make no sense in reality. This can be powerful and can lead to some very bad places—I'll describe one of mine later. These irrelevant thoughts can be far more than distractions, and lead to more than just poor decisions. In some instances, they can amount to a break with reality. No rational person would believe that a failed getaway attempt would be made better by taking hostages or that in some way snatching your child will convince the judge to give you custody, but criminals do similar things quite often. Not just criminals, either. Citizens, cops—maybe you—have done something that was monumentally stupid, but "seemed like a good idea at the time."

Behavioral looping is very common. Sometimes a person, especially a rookie, will focus on a single technique that IS NOT WORKING and he doesn't think to change it. It's very common in rookies to have them try to use the one technique that they really learned in training and just increase muscle and desperation when it doesn't work. Sometimes an officer or group of officers who were justified in using batons will run into a threat on which the baton doesn't work. Because focused blows with an impact weapon are the highest level of force below shooting, they stop there and just repeat the action, resulting sometimes in unnecessary injury. There is a chilling video available of the murder of Deputy Kyle Dinkheller taken from his dashboard camera. Even as the threat loads a rifle, Deputy Dinkheller stays locked in a verbal loop, repeating over and over, "Stop that," and "Stop loading that rifle!" He continues in that loop until he is shot.

As horrible as it sounds, as horrible as it is, all of these symptoms are survival responses for the worst case. You don't feel most pain (and neither does the threat. Pain-compliance locks and nerve points won't work). If you get cut or bitten, there is less bleeding. When animals evolved this reaction, it wasn't about being mugged; it was about being mauled by a lion or a bear. Situations where freezing, silence and not bleeding much are better survival strategies than trying to apply a nifty fingerlock or spinning kick of doom.

In 2003, a handful of us were pulled aside to put together a class for corrections officers who were going to have new duties outside the jail such as court officers and high-risk transports. We had everything: Sim guns (a real Glock that fires sub-caliber marking rounds) inert OC, foam batons, training Tasers, armor for the bad guys, and a modular training area.

The deputies would go into a scenario with a minimal briefing, e.g. "You're walking across the park by the courthouse," and sent into a situation that could be anything from a medical emergency to a lost child to a baby held hostage.

The class turned out to be a laboratory for adrenaline effects. Most of the students were veteran jailers. Many had hundreds of brawls under their belts. Many had not really experienced an adrenaline rush in years. Most were not "gunfighters."

We saw people adrenaline loop—some that had trouble drawing from level three holsters (that have two straps and an internal block) shot after the scenario was over because they had locked onto the *idea*. One turned and fired at a target that had been gone for several seconds but had just entered his conscious awareness. Many, when describing the scene after the scenario, added details that weren't there like descriptions of the reporter's microphone when the role player had had an empty hand.

At the academy, we were told one of the big mysteries of law enforcement: When criminals are shot several times, they usually get caught hundreds of yards away, climbing fences. When officers get shot, they curl up and die. I solved it in this training when I saw an officer shot in a scenario throw his hands up and say, "Ya got me!"

I was screaming, "Don't you dare die, you sonofabitch! Get back in the fight! You aren't dead until I say you're dead!" But I realized that this was the key. For most of us, the last time we were "shot" was playing cops-n-robbers as a kid. If you get shot playing cops-n-robbers, you curl up and die—*unless you're a cheater*. Cops were good kids. They don't cheat. The mind searches for the last time they were shot and they do what good kids do. They die.

An image: After a scenario that lasted probably two minutes and involved a lot of yelling and a single trigger pull, the officer was gasping for breath, hands on his knees, shaking and sweating. "Sarge, I feel like I'm going to cry and I want to puke. Is that normal?" That is perfectly normal.

There is an optimal stage of adrenalization. There is a point, you know it when you feel it, when you are on your game. You're alert, ready. Bruce Siddle, author of *Sharpening the Warrior's Edge*, has listed stages of adrenalization and indexed them by heart rate (as more stress hormones go into your system, the heart beat goes up). He states that around 115-145 BPM reaction time and fighting skills are maximized. Knowing this number won't help you a damn bit.

Different Cocktails

The predator versus the victim. As we've mentioned, the predator chooses the time and the place. One of the side effects is that the predator can manage his own level of arousal. It's subconscious, but the predator will work himself up or work himself down to that 115-145 BPM range. The victim? The victim will be at normal until the first contact and then will shoot off the chart, into the clumsy, frozen, perceptually-altered territory already mentioned.

It's not lightning. The hormones are released into the bloodstream, ergo it takes one heartbeat for the effects to kick in. If an effective response has been conditioned, the victim can get in one strike/action in that time. The beauty of this reflexive counterattack strategy is that it is not what the predator was expecting...which can kick his heartbeat off the chart and level the playing field.

Male and female adrenaline curves. In general, men get a big surge of adrenaline early that dissipates fairly quickly. Women have a much slower build up and a longer cool down time. Hence, a man will be ready to go berserk (or freeze) as soon as the engagement starts and a woman will be able to think clearly for several minutes before she hits her "deer in the headlights" mode.

This is easier to use offensively. If the threat is male, the longer you can put off the encounter, the less adrenalized and dangerous he will be. If the threat is female, the quicker you can end it, the less danger you will be in.

You can see this effect in arguments between spouses. The argument heats up, the man gets angry and goes for a walk, slamming the door behind him. A few minutes later, maybe a half hour, and he's calmed down. He's ready to talk; it was all silly anyway...blah, blah, blah. He comes home ready to talk just when his wife is hitting peak anger. He hardly knows what hit him.

The professional. With enough exposure, it is possible to become inured to certain types of violence. I know violence in my setting very well. I've literally had hundreds of jailhouse brawls, dozens of cell extractions, dealt with weapons and groups and ambushes several times.

Many years ago, there was a guy in a cell screaming threats. He was on drugs—either meth or PCP—and/or he was psychotic. I opened the door, spun him around, swept his feet, and knelt on his elbow and neck. It all took about a second, maybe two. The officer who followed me in, a rookie, looked at my free hand and whispered, "Sarge didn't even spill his coffee." I looked down and sure enough, a full coffee cup (it was a travel mug with a lid, this isn't a Jackie Chan movie). I took a sip while he put the handcuffs on. That was when I realized it was just a job.

Because I am used to that type of violence in that environment, I do have access to the fine and complex motor skills. I can make things work consistently that a rookie or a martial arts master cannot. However, if the situation changes, I start over. In 2002, because of knee surgery, I was assigned to be the shooter for the CERT instead of being in the stack (the line of officers making the entry) where I belong. Shooting, most of it came back: the tunnel vision, tachypsychia, and irrelevant thoughts.

The chemical cocktail makes most people more dangerous. It often makes trained fighters *less* dangerous. It increases strength, short-term speed, and lowers pain tolerance...all good things. It *decreases* skill sets and fine and complex motor skills. Fine and complex motor skills only apply to trained fighters. Untrained people are going to flail anyway and the hormone dump makes flailing more efficient. Trained people will often be forced to flail, eroding their efficiency.

Marc MacYoung, in *The Professional's Guide to Ending Violence Quickly,* said that you can see a shudder when the adrenaline hits. I haven't seen that. He then went on to describe three reactions to the chemical cocktail and these I have seen.

Some people get big, red, and loud. Their face flushes; they swell up and try to intimidate with size and voice. They are trying to intimidate,

---

Shock and Stupidity

Shock is the "inadequate perfusion of bodily tissue with blood and oxygen." In a very real way, shock is what kills people. Either the various organs don't get enough blood or the blood they do get has inadequate oxygen. Bleeding to death is hemorrhagic shock. Heart attack causes cardiogenic shock. Fainting is psychogenic shock.

EMTs are taught that one of the earliest signs of shock is agitation or nervousness. Far more often than I've seen agitation, I've noticed another symptom and it applies to shock, hypothermia, dehydration, hunger, sleep deprivation, and stress hormones: People tend to get really stupid ideas and then become extremely stubborn about them. This shows up in the behavioral loop, especially in the inability to see that the present action is not working and the resistance to changing the action.

---

pure and simple. They have more in common with the Monkey Dance than predatory violence. They are usually not a problem.

Small, white, and pale indicates a threat in a pretty advanced stage of adrenalization. His blood has pooled to his center and he is on the edge of panic. If something sets him off, he will go frantically insane. He will hurt you, much like a cornered animal.

Some go "flat" when the adrenaline hits. They seem emotionless, alert. Eyes widen into a thousand-yard stare. In general, they are experienced with the adrenaline state and can and will hurt you. They will retain a large percentage of skill. They make ugly opponents. On the good side, of the three types, these are the ones that can still communicate. You can talk to them.

Levels of Hormonal Stimulation

Bruce Siddle, in *Sharpening the Warrior's Edge*, has put together an excellent analysis of the various levels of "adrenalization." What follows is a simplification of his work, concentrating on what it feels like and how it affects your performance. In a later chapter, I'll address how to deal with the phenomenon (*See* Section 3.4).

For our purposes, there are four levels of stimulation:

Normal. Your day-to-day mind and body. Often not very alert or prepared for intense, violent action. When attacked in this state of mind, there is often a freeze as you adjust to what is happening. Your mind here will want to understand the situation before acting, which takes precious time if you are taking damage.

Optimal. There is a level of arousal where you are alert, engaged and physically ready to meet a challenge. This is where you mentally set yourself when preparing to spar—this is what "psyching up" is aiming for. Maximum perception, best reaction time, alert, and capable of planning and making decisions. Often, the skin of someone in this state is pink and has a healthy look.

Bad. Beyond the optimal state, you get into the signs and symptoms mentioned above. Physical and mental skills are seriously degraded. Most people in this state will be visibly pale.

Horrible. An absolute state of physical and often mental freezing. Sometimes associated with loss of bladder and bowel control.

Evolutionarily, this adrenalization response is a GOOD thing. Everything listed under the Bad and Horrible categories are advantages when faced with a carnivorous predator. No amount of technique (fine and complex motor skills) will drive a lion off; but a flailing (Gross Motor Activity, GMA), focused (tunnel vision), repetitive (behavioral loop) attack *might*.

Vasoconstriction in the extremities decreases the amount of bleeding from bites to arms, legs, and head. Desensitization to pain is a godsend when you are being eaten. Lastly, at the highest levels of arousal, a complete freeze (especially with bowel evacuation) is one of the few things that might convince a lion or bear that you are *dead*. If the predator is not hungry, it may "save you for later" and you *may* live.

This response is the bane of self-defense instructors. The annoying truth is that untrained people fight better under the chemical cocktail and trained people fight worse.

An untrained person in deep fear will respond to a human attack like the attack of a carnivorous animal. At the Bad level, they will flail; but if flailing is all they know how to do, they have no skill to lose. The focus and repetition and the ability to ignore pain can make them more efficient and dedicated fighters. Many of the mental and memory distortions, even the intrusive thoughts, may serve to keep the conscious mind from interfering. The body has a genetically programmed plan that has worked better than any alternatives for many millennia of lethal predatory assaults. It does not want the untested brain to interfere.

The trained person approaches combat in a completely different way. Using awareness of what the threat and other potential threats are doing (compromised by sensory distortion), the trained fighter makes or chooses a plan (compromised by cognitive distortion) and acts with a complex motor skill, coordinating the feet, hips, and arms (lost as the body switches to GMA), sometimes relying on finger dexterity or extreme precision (also compromised by GMA restriction).

The trained fighter loses more largely because he has more to lose, but also because he uses techniques designed and trained for the Optimal level of arousal. When the physiology is kicked into the higher, more animalistic ranges, the trained fighter is often unprepared.

section 3.4: adapting to the chemical cocktail

It is critical that you understand that there are different internal paths for dealing with the sudden dump of stress hormones and that they are dependent on time and fear, not on you. You don't get to choose.

I'm going to try to describe the situations and give advice for each type. The range in time is TIME, as in discretionary time, as in you see it coming, versus NO TIME.

The range in fear is from SCARED (the Bad level of stress response) to TERRIFIED (the Horrible level). If you can hit the Optimal level the first time out, you don't need my advice.

	SCARED Adrenaline is high; perception, coordination and thinking will be impaired.	TERRIFIED Frozen, incapable of moving.
NO TIME You are taking damage; the incident is happening.	NO TIME/SCARED As damage increases, your ability to respond is impaired. Responses are often inefficient.	NO TIME/TERRIFIED Taking damage and mentally or physically curling up in a ball. Must break the freeze by acting.
TIME You have seconds or minutes to plan or change the context or act first.	TIME/SCARED Breath control, centering to focus well enough to make a plan and act on it.	TIME/TERRIFIED Deer in the headlights, staring at harm as it comes to you. Imperative to recognize and break the freeze, then control through breathing, centering,

Different levels of fear interact with the amount of time available to limit your options to respond or dictate what must happen before you even can respond.

TIME/SCARED: When someone threatens you but you are pretty confident you can handle it, you'll get some serious adrenaline but you probably won't freeze. This is the best of the bad situations. This is also where all of the things you are taught in class work. Breathe, slow and deep, in through your nose and subtly out through your mouth. Center. In this context, that means feel your belly/hips, especially if you have been taught to strike or move with hip action, and check your footing. One of my favorite fighters, Mac, will say, "You let your energy get too high." What he is saying is that some people go up on the balls of their feet for mobility, but go too far, sacrificing balance and power. Clear the spine—shift your hips, shoulders, and head a little to stretch by twisting.

Keep your hands close, preferably touching something or lightly moving. I put one under the opposite elbow, splinting my ribs, and the other, usually stroking my jaw. It keeps you from visibly shaking (and neither you nor the threat needs to see you shake).

If you can hear your heartbeat, slow it down. It does work.

Personally, I have the breathing down to a single "here we go again" sigh. Then I check my footing, feeling the muscles tighten in my legs, and clear the spine. To the threat, I look both bored and ready. I have never had an experienced fighter, who saw me clear the spine, keep the challenge up.

TIME/TERRIFIED—LONG TERM: I've never experienced this—bed-wetting terror but with time before the threat becomes tangible. When this happens it usually takes a long-term program of terrorizing the victim. Subconsciously, operant conditioning principles have been used to convince the victim that resistance equals pain. You'll see this in victims of serious abuse, people whose parents have turned them into complete victims. You'll also see it in old films of the death camps. Maybe it's not so rare after all. It can turn into a kind of hopeless resignation, just because the human body can't keep the fear up for very long.

For many of these victims, it will not occur to them to act. If it does, it can occur at a crisis point or an objectively safe time. Be aware that there is no *subjective* safe time. Someone who has been in this situation may feel that everything is a trap and every movement or even thought is watched.

A crisis point is a moment of damage or imminent damage. It becomes a NO TIME/TERRIFIED.

There is discretionary time built into this scenario—time to plan and gather resources, and act. The victim must act. She or he has to get out of the situation and out of the cycle or it will continue to escalate. This is less about controlling the chemical cocktail than it is about choosing those times when it is abated. Timing, in the self-defense sense, becomes critical: You act when you can get away with it. You have a go button (e.g., "when the threat goes into town for groceries."). When the go button hits, you move. Decisively.

This is easy to say, but I'd be bullshitting if I implied it was easy to do. In long-term abuse, in prisoner of war situations and in concentration camps, the people in power diligently used their power to alter the victim's will—in essence, to edit their story, their identity, to that of a character who wouldn't or couldn't act.

TIME/TERRIFIED—IMMEDIATE: I remember two incidents, both from a long time ago. Once I was reading outside on a summer day and my sister said, "Rory! Don't move!" and pointed down. A four-foot rattlesnake was coiled under my chair.

Later that same year, a group of older kids with knives were circling me, talking about how they were going to cut me open, and I couldn't move. I wish I could finish these war stories with some brilliant strategy. With the rattler, I jumped about twelve feet in the air. With the kids, I didn't die because they didn't want to kill me.

The hardest part about being terrified is that your brain freezes. Unless the idea to act crosses your mind, you have no chance of acting. It's reflexive and obvious, but true. This is the hardest to train for and deal with because you don't even have a flinch reaction to break the immobility.

In order to train, you will need someone you can trust to be ruthless and unpredictable. The key is to trigger this state so that you can recognize it. If you use only one method to trigger the state, you will start to adapt to the training method, not to the state. Following are some drills that will trigger a panic reaction in some people:

If you have not already trained to inure yourself to face contact, start at the upper end of the spectrum—give your ruthless partner permission to slap you when you aren't expecting it.

If you do not practice contact training, have your partner hit you with a good headshot during sparring. Though I can't recommend hard head contact as a long-term training method (microconcussions are a bitch), the feeling after a good head shot, with the roaring ears and dream-like feeling, is very much like being frozen.*

Have your partner unexpectedly introduce a knife. For most people, the flash of steel when they are expecting just a regular class can make them freeze.

If you know of buttons that make you freeze—words, a scenario, or a true phobia—introduce it.

If you recognize the state, you have a much better chance of breaking it. As soon as you realize you are frozen, do something; act. It doesn't have to be a big act. Breathing is good enough. "Inhale,"

---

*It's not unpleasant or even scary to be frozen. You will often have the illusion of good, reasonable thought. One of my junior deputies, who stood and watched while another deputy was injured, denied he froze. "No, Sarge, I wasn't frozen. I saw everything. I even knew he was going to get hurt. It was like he was in slow motion. Just for whatever reason, I decided not to do anything. It made sense at the time." The state is almost dream-like.

you tell yourself, and you breathe in. The first goal is to get your body to do something (anything) your mind has directed it to do. That breaks the first layer. If your survival is not dependent on hiding, scream. A good, lung-cleansing scream really helps focus. Then plan, and act. You have just turned this from a TERRIFIED to a SCARED situation.

NO TIME/SCARED: In NO TIME situations, you are taking damage before you are even consciously aware of the attack. Your body will be calling the shots on how much of the chemical cocktail gets dumped in your system. This situation must be dealt with and trained for in advance. The key components will be contact response training, followed by hormone management and technique training.

The timeline will go:

Sudden attack (stimulus).

Response (your high percentage reflex technique).

Simultaneous hormone cascade (which will put you in SCARED or TERRIFIED level and it won't be your choice) AND first evaluation.

Cognitive control. If your Stimulus/Response training was good, you've already hit him or broken away and created space. Because of the hormone cascade, you will now have to remind yourself what to do next. "Right, right—I'm supposed to hit him again."

Hit him again.

At this stage, good training will kick in. Your body has seen that the plan/training has worked and will quit trying to freeze you. It is imperative that the training work and that you not be given unrealistic expectations. If you have been taught that a threat will go down to a thigh kick and he doesn't, the difference between what is happening and what is expected may cause a second freeze.

Only steps 4 and 5 of this protocol are decided in the event. The contact/response, ability to actually fight, and expectations of what the fight will be like are established in training long before the incident.

NO TIME/TERRIFIED: The dynamics of this situation are similar, except you are frozen. There is little good advice I can give you except that you must recognize the frozen state and force yourself to act, as described above. The difference is that you will be taking damage the whole time. The longer it takes for you to unfreeze, the less likely you will be physically able to respond properly.

Training and Experience

Experience is no substitute for training.

Training is no substitute for experience.

The one huge advantage in dealing with a true ambush, a real NO TIME situation, is that I have done it before. I remember that the damage was cosmetic and that there was blood dripping down my face, but I was thinking, "I've been injured worse than this in class. I've been hurt worse by my friends. MY WIFE HITS HARDER THAN YOU!"

Not that my wife abuses me; she's a *karateka* and we spar.

Experience is funny. We think that the more experience we have, the more confidant we will be in the future. For most things, that's true. In violence, for me, experience has given me a deeper understanding of the stakes I fight for and a profound respect for the role that luck plays. I am far less confident than I was in my twenties, yet far more competent.

There is a comfortable illusion that with enough repetitions, drills, or scenarios, real life will be "just like training." Real life is the only thing that is "just like" real life.

Training is also important. What would be the point of breaking through the freeze, regaining conscious control of the moment and taking the initiative, if you don't know what to do?

As if breaking the freeze wasn't trouble enough, there's more. No matter how hard you have trained, how much you have studied, or how closely you have matched your training environment to the realities that you face, your body and primitive mind know that you have only been faking.

Training and planning are blueprints, nothing more. They are plans; they are stories that you tell yourself. You may truly believe that your new skill (new system, new plan) is the best way out of your situation—but your body knows one thing, too: What you are already doing hasn't gotten you killed yet.

In the moment, like breaking the freeze, you must force yourself to act. Once a few steps are taken on the new path and you *haven't* died, the primitive brain will ease up a bit.

As Lonnie Athens pointed out (*see* Richard Rhodes' *Why They Kill*), this is why change is hard. No matter how horrible and abusive one's past, no matter how desperately a change is needed or how obviously deadly the current course of action (or inaction) is, the primitive part of your brain wants to freeze or continue in a behavioral loop because it hasn't gotten you killed yet; and especially when death is in the air, it feels that any change could bring it on.

You can weaken this over time by changing a habit. Practice stepping off the blueprint. Take a class you know nothing about. Introduce yourself to strangers. Go to restaurants or vacation spots you've never been to before. Take a cold shower. One aspect of the identity story is that we quickly classify ourselves. "I'm the kind of person who would never do *that*." Finding these sticking points and breaking them is one of the key small habits that can both help you adapt in an unexpected emergency and make you more resilient in recovery.

section 3.5: the context of violence

Violence always happens in a specific place, at a specific time and between people. In the sterile *dojo* environment it is easy to concentrate on the physical actions of assault and forget that action always comes from somewhere. Every so often we play a game in my class. We set out a bench as a bus seat and have the new students one by one sit in the seat. I'll put on the slimiest attitude I can fake and slowly approach the sitting student, ogling her (or him, it creeps guys out too) then slowly drawing my hand along their shoulders.

It's a martial arts class doing a scenario. Most students push my hand away and give me a ferocious stare. They are dealing with the action, being assertive but not aggressive—all good stuff.

I then have Roz, a more senior student, take the chair as one of the new students gets to role-play the slimy bad guy. As the new student touches her shoulder, Roz shrieks, "Get your hands off me you filthy pervert!" and the new student jerks away, stunned.

With voice alone, Roz attacked the context. Certain types of predators are like cockroaches—they don't like light. They don't like attention. On the bus or train, every eye would suddenly be riveted to this guy. Often, one or two men will start moving forward (I've seen this in real encounters; but to be fair, I was always one of the people moving forward; perhaps there would have been no action without me starting).

The threat was looking for a world where people are polite even to assholes, and if he got lucky and found someone too meek to even meet his eyes, he might have found his victim. He does not want to be seen and remembered by dozens of witnesses.

The context of violence can be divided into place, time, and people.

section 3.6: violence happens in places

There are certain categories of places that account for a huge percentage of violence out there. It is the people who congregate there that make the place dangerous, but the place is what you will see first.

Violence happens where people get their minds altered. Drugs and alcohol at the most basic level change the way people think and act. Honestly, smell is the only way to tell a drunk person from a really stupid one. Only a stupid person or a drunk would think that groping a young woman in front of a bar full of witnesses was a good idea. Or after being rejected think that getting a shotgun from the car was a good response.

Other drugs such as PCP, crack, and meth can put the threat into a frenzied, manic state where thoughts of killing and suicide and fun all seem to blend together. DO NOT try to understand a chemically-altered mind from the context of your normal one. I have been very successful, on occasion, at calming down really methed-up freaks. I've also had them explode into violence, decide I was a higher order being in their tribal religion, try to drive their own head into a brick wall at full speed, and explain that they were all scratched up because they figured out that if they stripped naked and ran through a blackberry patch it would cure their addiction.

It didn't work, in case you were wondering.

Drugs and alcohol are also high-volume cash businesses and draw more than their share of armed robberies, which can always go bad. Areas of cities with high drug crime will also have high violent crime as groups and individuals fight for "market share" in a business where there is no recourse to contract lawyers or police.

Violence happens where young men gather in groups. Lots of violence, minor and major, is based on the Monkey Dance or Group Monkey Dance models. The Monkey Dance is primarily a young male phenomenon, as older men have usually established their status. Young men, still struggling to establish status or identity, are extreme risks for MD attacks. A reputation for violence is very valuable in establishing status with this group. It does not need to be real ability, just a reputation. Some seek to gain that reputation in the safest possible way. This is the bully dynamic, gaining a reputation while exclusively targeting safe victims. If you wander into this environment as an unknown quantity with no reputation, you will be examined and, if deemed "safe," a low status group member may try to challenge or provoke you. It will likely happen in full view of the group, partially because the threat wants witnesses to his dominance ploy, but also because the threat will feel safer with friends near at hand.*

The Group Monkey Dance is another situation and the group can be male, female, or mixed. The trigger for the assault may have nothing to do with you—the group could just move down the street, throwing bottles and mauling anyone who doesn't run. Or it could have everything to do with a perceived insult to the group or a higher ranked member.

Violence happens where territories are in dispute. Lots of gang violence, lots of military violence—let's just call it social violence—happens in places where two or more groups are trying to run things. Even a gang with undisputed control of an area is vying with the good citizens and the cops, resulting in a combat mentality, which can turn

---

* Not a sure bet, but the group often won't get involved. The very lowest members vying for status with outsiders doesn't threaten the *group's* identity. If the low-ranking member loses, it's a source of amusement.

to violence quickly. We focus on crimes here, but war zones are the classic "social violence" milieu, where two or more armed groups are vying for control. They produce similar kinds of violence for similar reasons, including "collateral damage" killings of noncombatants and bystanders.

Don't think of territory wholly as space. True, people identify with their territory and will fight for their homes, their "turf," or their "hood." But they are fighting for their identity, not the piece of ground. Violence is so psychologically damaging, not because of the physical damage but because of the attack on self-image, the attack on one's identity.

People fight and kill to defend *imaginary* territory—respect and honor, symbols, membership in a group. They are not fighting to defend their lives but only to defend the way that they see themselves.

Do not mistake this as an artificial or weak drive. We revere martyrs who died for a religion. We make statues of people who risked their lives to plant a flag. In each case, they gave up their lives for something abstract. The exact same drive moves a gangbanger to kill another for the color of a scarf. It is all in defense of the story.

Predatory violence happens in lonely places. Attacks happen where the predator believes he is unlikely to be disturbed and witnesses are rare. A sudden assault with intent to murder, rape, or rob is a planned action. The predator has taken care to choose a place *and* time that benefit him. Often, he has lured the victim to a more private place or charmed his way into the victim's home. The lonelier the place, the more time and more noise the predator can afford to make.

The secondary crime scene. The first crime scene is where the initial assault and abduction took place. The secondary crime scene is where the human predator takes his victims so that he can spend more time and have greater privacy. Assault, robbery, and even murder don't necessarily take a lot of time. If the predator needs time and privacy, it is for rape and torture. It is my opinion that you would generally have a better chance of survival driving your car off a cliff with your entire family inside than to allow yourself to be driven to the predator's secondary crime scene.

Home invasions are crimes where a criminal or criminals deliberately choose a house they know to be occupied and enter in force to rob, rape, and/or murder. Home invasion crimes have many of the elements of a secondary crime scene. Your home is private and secure, exactly what a predatory criminal may want. In addition, threats against family members can be used as leverage to force cooperation with the predator. This cooperation will not be to the victim's benefit.

If someone holds a gun to your child's head and orders you to go to the garage and get duct tape and a hammer, you have two choices. (1) If you run from the garage and call the police from the neighbor's, the invader will have to choose whether to stay or run. He may kill your child, or decide not to risk the murder charge. (2) If you cooperate and return with the duct tape and hammer, what is he going to do with them? Whatever it is, he will do it to your child and make you watch, and then he will do it to you.

For analysis and tactical advice on some of the most savage crimes, I recommend Sanford Strong's *Strong on Defense*.

Fishing for victims is different. Whereas predatory assaults happen in lonely places, fishing for victims can happen in crowds. The predator is looking for an easy mark. There are a handful of victim personalities and the predator hunts for them. Using eye contact, body language, and proximity, the predator sees who will back down without eye contact, who will pretend an inappropriate touch didn't happen, who will try to curry favor with those they see as strong.

It is especially appealing for predators to work areas where drugs and alcohol are common. Alcohol makes you stupid. For some people that means that violence is more likely. For others, the impaired judgment means that they are much easier victims. Think how many severely drunk women have been victimized on college campuses.

Someone is going to read this and think, "I have a right to go anywhere I want. Just because something is dangerous doesn't take away my rights." Let's get this over with now. Defending yourself is not and never has been about rights—rights are those things that the civilized members of society agree everyone deserves. When you hit the ground and taste blood in your mouth, when a steel-toed boot slams your head into a curb, when a knife slips under the waistband of your skirt and a hand is wrapped around your throat, the civilized agreement on how people should be treated is not an issue.

On one level, self-defense is about not getting damaged. On another level, it's about not waking up sweating and screaming; being able to have a trusting, intimate relationship; not feeling your palms sweat whenever you see an open closet. Even if you "win," even if you come through completely unscathed, you can still suffer, sometimes for years. T. Rose writes, "Self-defense is not having your lifestyle changed for you."

It's better to avoid than to run; better to run than to de-escalate; better to de-escalate than to fight; better to fight than to die. The very essence of self-defense is a thin list of things that might get you out alive when you are already screwed.

section 3.7: violence happens in time

There is a difference between *violence* and the *threat* of violence. That distance is time. If the violence is *happening*, if the gun is coming online, the knife is plunging at your belly, or something cracks over the back of your head—you need to be moving. The *threat of violence* is a gift, someone communicating to you that they intend or are considering using violence, BUT THEY HAVEN'T YET. Someone threatening to hurt you has given you information and precious time. Use the time.

The Threat of Violence: You Have Time

Lieutenant Webb, an instructor at the academy long ago, used to say, "No intelligent man has ever lost a fight to someone who said, 'I'm gonna kick your ass!'" Those words were the signal and the license to prepare yourself. Leave. Get a weapon. Call the police. Call some friends. Find cover. Do whatever you need to do to stay healthy.

Use of discretionary time is one of the most valuable concepts in emergency response and one of the hallmark differences between a

> ## Hostage Situations
>
> Potentially, hostage takings can be one of the most drawn-out and complex situations that fall under the "Threat of Violence" category. A hostage situation is about one or more armed threats holding you and/or others, using the threat of violence to get what they want.

veteran and a rookie. Discretionary time is time to think, time when information is coming in and you have options but you do not need to move just yet. It is time to plan. A rookie medic runs to the car wreck, the veteran stops and checks for fallen power lines. The rookie officer jumps into the fight, the veteran looks at the spectators first, checks his resources and needs and then makes a decision as to what will work best.

If you have time to plan, even a second, use it. If you do not, if you are taking damage, you need to be moving, to be running or fighting. While you are taking damage, all thoughts of planning or trying to figure out what is happening or why take time. Time is damage.

Types of Hostage Takers

Dumb ones. Most commonly, a person committing a felony gets caught or trapped and feels that the best chance of getting away is to take a hostage as a bargaining tool. This is a bad idea. The moron has just traded a (for instance) First Degree Robbery charge for Robbery and Felony Kidnapping charges and anything else the prosecuting attorney can tack on. (Unless you are up on the arcane ins and outs of criminal law as they apply to felons in that jurisdiction, let the Crisis Negotiation Team (CNT) bring up this point.)

Nutballs. People suffering from mental illness may take hostages. Statistically, it will be a member of his own family. The actual act of taking hostages and how the threat acts will be based on a rigid internal logic. You have to analyze your relationship with that person from their point of view. Get them talking. Let them vent. Be prepared for things to go bad quickly.

Fanatics and Extremists. Contrary to Hollywood portrayals, these are not well-trained teams of cold-blooded sociopaths. They are angry people who want to make a statement. Their very fanaticism gives you a good starting point for personalizing yourself. Listen. Pay attention.

People who want to die. Suicide by cop is an interesting phenomenon. The threat wants to die, doesn't quite have the courage to kill himself, and plans to force the police to do it. Taking hostages is one way to make sure that a large number of well-armed cops show up quickly. This one will probably get messy, but the threat usually has enough guilt issues that they will be reluctant to add a murder to the list. Not always.

Disposable terrorists. With the exception of the plane take-overs on 9/11, this hasn't happened in the Unites States yet, but it is possible. Consider it a heads-up from Russia. This will be a large group of heavily-armed people who will attempt to take a large group of hostages in a defensible place. They will cow the hostages by brutally and visibly killing anyone who is likely to resist or shows any leadership ability, such as by comforting crying children. They may also torture and rape to make the hostages too afraid to resist. In the past, they have wired the hostages or the hostage holding area with bombs. They will drag out the negotiations—not because they want anything and they have no wish for any of the hostages to live—the disposable terrorist wants maximum media coverage and a chance to fortify his position. The more hostages and the more officers he kills, the better his terrorist organization can use the event for propaganda. Run if you can; run early and often. There are no high-percentage survival techniques for this situation.

Process predators. This is a special case. This threat does not want something from someone else. He wants to rape, torture, and kill for the longest time and with the greatest privacy he can arrange. Remember the entry on secondary crime scenes and home invasion crimes (*See* Section 3.6)? There is no good result of a violent criminal wanting to be alone with you.

Some things to know. In a hostage situation, except for the predator scenario and the disposables, generally the longer it lasts the better. Most people—even dangerous, violent people—can't kill "cold." They need to work themselves up, need the adrenaline. Adrenaline is hard to keep up. As they come down off their edge it will be harder and harder for them to act violently until they get angry or scared again.

Of the hostage-taker types mentioned above, they all want something. With the exception of the predator, the disposable terrorist and sometimes the nutballs, what they want is not served by killing you. The dumb one would tack on a murder charge. The nutball generally wants help and to be understood. The fanatic wants a message to get out and knows that the message will be obscured if innocents are killed. The suicidal one just wants to die, not to kill. The predator and the DT are the only ones who plan to kill you as part of the operation.

The 9/11 hijackings were similar to the disposable terrorist model and used the DT methods for cowing the hostages, but the 9/11 hijacking was never truly a hostage situation. The terrorists would have preferred empty planes. The passengers, in fact, were one of the few things that could screw with their plans, as they did on flight UA93. Those passengers, realizing they were going to die, fought back.

Why didn't the passengers on the other planes? Because in the vast majority of hijackings before 9/11, the passengers weren't killed. They weren't killed because doing so would have obscured the message. When killings happened in terrorist attacks, it was a bombing or a shooting. Kidnapping and trying to hold large groups of people for the purpose of killing them is difficult and inefficient. This changed, I believe, as the focus for international terrorism changed from causing terror and political change in the target country to increasing financial contributions from sympathizers. Not so long ago, the terrorist preferring to die to send a message (there had always been a few *willing*) was more myth than reality. It still is—even at Beslan, the terrorists had an escape strategy—but as terrorism becomes big business receiving huge donations, there is far more incentive to mold the impressionable mind into a somewhat less survival-oriented puppet.

In a very real sense, 9/11 was never a hostage taking. It was a mobile bombing. It very much followed the dynamics of the GMD, and each of the hijackers established their loyalty to the group with their deaths.

Even if the goal is not to kill the hostages, the situation is still very dangerous. If you have a group of scared or angry armed men and a group of panicked hostages, the chances of violence erupting are very high.

If the hostage takers are a group, watch the dynamics—leadership, morale, level of organization. Because they can cover for each other's fatigue and stupidity, opportunities to act will be less common. Purely because of numbers, fighting will be riskier.

With an individual, look for mental illness, motivation, drug or alcohol use, and fatigue. Mental illness or motivation may give you the hooks you need to personalize yourself. Drugs and fatigue may give you the opening you need to act.

Tactics. Personalize yourself. It is much harder to kill someone you know than a stranger. If at all possible, make sure the hostage takers know your name and face. If conversations happen, look for common areas of interest, but don't be phony. The goal is to make it harder to see you as an outsider. This is one reason why a drawn out hostage situation is more likely to be resolved without killing—as the criminals get to know the hostages as people, it becomes harder to kill them. Sound as calm as possible. Listen. Try to control the *rate, tone, pitch* and *volume* of your voice. Low, slow, calm, and soothing. You are trying to become a person in the eyes of the threat.

Empathy not sympathy. It is very useful to try to understand the threat's point of view, that will help you personalize; but DO NOT get caught up in it. The Stockholm Syndrome has been overplayed, but victims do get emotionally bonded with the threat. For both of them, it is usually the single most intense event of their lives. Be aware of that, because if your "Go" button (*See* Section 6.2) gets pushed, you will need to act resolutely, decisively, ruthlessly, and immediately...and personalizing can work both ways.

The above two points do not apply to the disposable terrorists. They have read the same manuals as the hostage negotiators, the SWAT teams, and the Hostage Survival Instructors. They will recognize the tactics and they will kill you for trying. This makes it a critical skill to tell, as early as possible, if the men with the guns are in this category.

If you get an opportunity to leave, leave. EVEN IF IT MEANS LEAVING YOUR FAMILY BEHIND. Your information from the inside may make a huge difference in tactical operations. In a home invasion, leaving will force the threat to choose between staying, torturing, and murdering the family members he has left, or running before you can call the police. Or you can stay and be tortured and murdered in your turn, after watching your family go through it.

Do not let the hostage taker control you by threatening someone else. This applies especially to predators. Some will use you and will take delight in using you to provide the murder weapon or to be the one to tie up the first victim. Give some deep thought to where this falls as a "Go" button. But if they send you to get duct tape or a knife, even if they are holding a gun to your child's head, take the opportunity to leave. Force the threat to choose to run or stay. The worst thing he can do in a minute to your child will not approach what he will do to both of you if given your cooperation and a few hours.

Do not allow yourself to be tied, handcuffed, or moved to a secondary crime scene. Some experts disagree with this and suggest acquiescence. They believe, with justification, that a failed attempt to resist will cause the criminals to use greater force to maintain or establish control. My rationale for resisting is simply this: Once you are restrained, you are out of options. When and if it becomes appropriate or necessary to act, you will not be able to.

In general, respond to the situation as it is. Not to your fantasy (I bet I can kick the gun out of his hand) and not to your paranoia (he put the gun down and is pouring a drink—it must be a trap).

Acts of Violence: You Have No Time

Once the violence starts, it is too late to plan. Your options are limited. This is very simple. You either run or fight or hide.

Running. In Section 6.1, we'll discuss Escape and Evasion (E&E) as an important habit to develop. For now, remember that distance is your friend. Making distance is more likely to make someone miss with a handgun than any fancy evasive maneuvers.

Be sure to run to a safe place. Knowing where the safe places are and the safe routes to them is where the E&E habit pays off.

The statistics on misses are encouraging. Most people miss most of the time, even at extremely close range.

What the Pros Are Doing:

With the exception of the predator, where it is very unlikely the professionals have any idea you are in trouble, the police will respond to a hostage situation by:

- Evacuating the nearby area.

- Setting up an inner and outer perimeter.

- Preparing a tactical plan.

- Gathering intelligence on the layout, the threat and the hostages.

- Establishing or attempting to establish contact with the threat.

What YOU should do if the tactical team makes an entry:

- Hit the floor face first and cover the back of your neck with your interlaced fingers (so that they can see your hands as well as offering some protection).

- Follow all orders.

- Keep your hands visible.

- Expect to be treated like a threat—handcuffed, searched, and segregated—until the police have sorted out who is who and what is what.

Statistics on survivability are also good. Most people recover fully. Corollary—DO NOT LET YOUR IMAGINATION KILL YOU! If you are shot or stabbed, KEEP RUNNING! Do not curl up and die because that's what you've seen on TV. One soldier took over thirty rifle bullets and still carried two men to the helicopter. A criminal in Baton Rouge took ten .357 bullets to the head and chest, including a contact shot to the center of the chest, an armpit to armpit through-and-through, and a penetration of the skull. Even after that last shot, where the officer stated he looked into the hole he blew into the man's skull, the threat still managed to start to attack again. BE THAT DEDICATED.

If you just walked into a situation, the route you took in should be a safe one to take out.

Run early and often. If you walk into your local Stop 'n' Rob convenience store and see a guy with a gun by the counter...that's all you need. Run. Even if he says, "Stop!" Even if he says, "I won't hurt you." You do not need to investigate a little more thoroughly to see if running is really the right thing to do. This is a really stupid inclination that some people have that mystifies me. It's right up there with "I thought I heard a rattlesnake or something so I bent down to look under the log." Or looking for gas leaks with a match.

Hiding. Sometimes an option. Not in a small place or an open place, but if you are good at it or have scoped out some spots, it's worth a try. In a large victim pool, such as a workplace shooting, it is easy to be missed entirely. You can make finding hidey-holes part of your E&E habit.

Fighting. Of everything in this book, skill at fighting is the least likely to affect your survival in a sudden assault. It's better to avoid than to run; better to run than to de-escalate; better to de-escalate than to fight; better to fight than to die. This is covered more in Chapter 6.

To be perfectly clear, I am not talking about brawling, dueling, sparring, or martial arts. What you need falls more into the category of assassination techniques or explosive, overwhelming "blitz" attacks.

No one voluntarily faces a gun armed only with a sword, or faces a sword armed only with a knife, or faces a knife unarmed...but look at all the training that goes into that.

The very essence of self-defense is a thin list of things that might get you out alive when you are already screwed.

section 3.8: violence happens between people

Chapter 4 is about bad guys and predators in and of themselves. This section is about the dynamic between the attacker and the victim. It ties in very much to the places to avoid mentioned above.

If the threat is acting for social reasons and the person is in the same or similar social status, the aggressor will pick his dance partner based on an accurate, subconscious assessment of benefit and risk. Remember that in most cases the dynamic here is completely subconscious.

I worked casino security for about two years and was never jumped. I'm five foot nine and weighed 145 pounds. Thai, one of my partners, played college football and almost made the 49ers in open tryouts. Thai was big, fast, and in great shape. It seemed like he was getting swung on every couple of weeks. It took awhile to figure out what was happening. One glance at me and for the average Monkey Dancin' drunk it was obvious—he wins and his friends tease him about beating up on a little kid. He loses and he'll never live it down. He attacked the big football player, though, especially one who is really professional and will try not to injure him, he can count on scoring a big reputation, win or lose, with relatively little chance of getting hurt.

The choice of victim is heavily influenced by fear and, in a strange way, self-esteem. In a straight Monkey Dance, the aggressor will pick the person they perceive to be at their level. Remember how mom always told you that bullies are cowards? They choose people much weaker because that is the level of status they believe they belong in. They are afraid to tackle bigger targets.

In certain areas with a fairly well-organized hierarchy of thugs, reputation is very, very important. Since most of the thugs in the area will have friends, it is easier and safer to develop a reputation for ruthlessness, cruelty, or "being hard" on tourists or strangers. This is the dynamic behind some of the brutal attacks between strangers in public places. The aggressor has a huge advantage, not only in that he knows the attack is going to happen but because a stranger who is not aware of local customs will too often be in denial that the attack is even happening.

GMD violence happens most often when an outsider violates a territorial boundary, a local taboo, or interferes in group activities, such as crime. I realize I use animals as examples, but it works: We're animals. The dynamic in GMD is like a pack of dogs chasing sheep.

They may not be hungry dogs so they may not be out for the kill, but it's fun to make sheep run and cause pain. If the sheep happens to get shredded, it's not a big deal either. Sheep don't try to talk themselves out of these situations. They do occasionally fight and we did have a ram that drove off a coyote when I was a kid, but it was an especially aggressive and insane ram—something the people who successfully fight against groups also have in common.

My caution in the GMD is to not approach it as a problem between people, but as a very dangerous situation between predator and prey or pack predators versus lone stranger.

In the predator dynamic, the victim is a resource, pure and simple. The experienced predator has worked out his system to get what he wants as easily and safely as possible. We've discussed aspects of this before and will do so again.

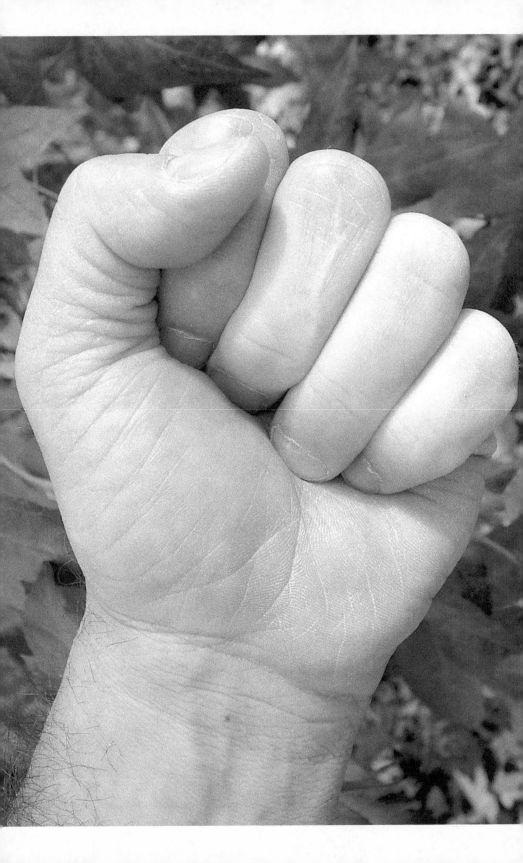

CHAPTER 4: PREDATORS

section 4.1: threats ain't normal folks

Almost all humans have a self-referencing test for effectiveness: If it works on me, it works. This is almost true. If it works on you, it will work on the majority of normal, sane people without drugs or alcohol in their systems who aren't really scared or really angry.

Our tactical team has this cool set of tools that are labeled "Less Lethal" technology. These are things like small bags of lead shot (called bean-bag rounds) or rubber bullets that are fired from a shotgun. When we first got them, I wanted to be shot with each of them (I'm a *rabid* self-referencer). My lieutenant said I was crazy, ordered me not to let anybody shoot me, and read us the statistics from the manufacturer. According to the manufacturer, these tools were destined to revolutionize our job.

Until we used them on bad guys. The first inmate we used bean-bag rounds on at relatively close range took four in the stomach and contemptuously batted the fifth out of the air with his hand. We wound up using the shotgun as a hand-to-hand weapon in the ensuing melee. We quit using that round.

Then the rubber bullets. I mention this in an essay in Chapter 7. Suffice to say that a "Less Lethal" munition that was rated to be safe at five feet blew a hole in a person at twenty feet, big enough for your thumb. We quit using that round, too.

If a threat is in full-survival mode, fighting for his life, he is not in the same state of mind that you were in when you said, "Ow! That wristlock really hurts! I'm going to learn that one good!"

Then throw drugs into the mix, drugs that can make the threat immune to the pain. Drugs that jump their metabolism off the chart. Drugs that completely remove any civilized conditioning they may have had. Drugs that allow them to apply more power than their tendons and bones can support.

Fist
Courtesy Kamilla Z. Miller

We had an inmate in custody who had cut open a baby with a tin can lid and raped the wound. If someone can do that, do you think he will hesitate at all before gouging your eye out or biting off a finger?

We had to take down an inmate who was running full force into a steel door again and again and again. We had to stop him before he killed himself. If he had turned that rage on us, if we had given him the time to focus on us, do you think any competition could have prepared us for that level of commitment? He wanted to die. He wasn't PREPARED to die, he WANTED it. There is a difference. I've twice gone into that situation with people who wanted to die but wanted to take someone with them when I didn't have my team to back me up. There may be a higher level of risk. I haven't seen it.

The question to ask isn't whether the technique worked in class—it's whether it would work if the person applying it was terrified and the person he was using it on was completely enraged, attacking in a frenzy and totally immune to pain.

The first real sociopath I met was in a maximum-security jail. Maybe I met dozens, actually, but this was the first I recognized. He'd been the inmate given the job of helping to keep clean the thirty-two-bed module I was supervising. He held that position throughout his trial. We talked often, but never about his case. He was intelligent and articulate. When he was eventually found guilty, he wanted to talk about it. I listened.

He was upset because the judge had not understood how his behavior was necessary. In each of the cases, he had politely asked the woman for sex first. His victims were the ones who had the effrontery to say "no." Of course he raped them. He honestly felt that asking first was commendable, going out of his way to be polite to a lower order of being—a woman. He'd only hurt the ones who fought. He couldn't let the word get out on the street that he'd let a woman hit him, so of course he had to kill her.

"You're a man," he said, "you understand, right?"

He had been raised to believe that as the oldest son everything was his by right and any resistance to that natural order had to be put down savagely. The end result was nearly fifty counts of rape, sodomy, kidnap, assault, and attempted murder.

There are two codas to this story:

First, four or five years later, his younger brother came through the system. I recognized the name and talked with the kid for a while. I said I'd known his brother. The kid said, "Yeah, they railroaded him. No way he could have done what they said he did, he has a bad back." The rapist had told me that he did it, but within the family the oldest boy was perfect and could do no wrong, despite any evidence or trail of shattered bodies.

Second, as I was writing this, I Googled the sociopath's name. He's looking for a female pen pal on meet-an-inmate.com. He's looking for someone special, looking forward to making her smile, and promises "no games."

Life Behind Bars...

One of the most frustrating things for people who truly want to change the world is that users, which includes almost all criminals, can twist almost anything to serve their purposes no matter how noble the original intent. The provisions of the FMLA (Family Medical Leave Act) have been abused to get free vacation time; jails have become health stations and resting places for hustlers; workout equipment intended to promote health and alleviate boredom is used to make a harder, more violent and more fit convict; drug treatment programs have become places to make connections and ways to avoid doing time, getting many of the benefits of jail without the inconveniences.

To live a criminal lifestyle is to become a skilled exploiter. There is no program so noble, or (as yet) so well-designed, that a skilled exploiter can not only avoid changing, but actually abuse it to become enabling.

---

section 4.2: the types of criminal

I work with criminals. I know them. This will be a slight departure from the subject of violence, but it is critical. Much like any other assumption, people usually have experience with one of the three types of criminals and try to generalize it to the others. It is a mistake. It is a mistake in self-defense and it is possibly a greater mistake when people try to write law or policy to deal with crime.

People who made a mistake. These are relatively rare. Every so often someone who was raised with a good sense of right and wrong will do something illegal. The good sense of right and wrong is the key...a stable, two-parent family and all that helps but good people come from every background, and some of them make mistakes.

Only this group will be truly ashamed. Only this group is affected by the jail system enough not to come back. If they are charged with a violent crime, it will be in a Monkey Dance or from a loss of control under the influence of drugs and alcohol. There is a possibility that someone engaging in legitimate self-defense might be charged with a crime and he would fall under this category, but I haven't seen that.

Every sympathetic character you have seen in prison dramas falls into this category. Almost all policies and the very concept of rehabilitation are based on a belief that this is the "average" criminal. Someone who made "bad choices," someone who made a mistake.

These guys are rare as hell. Due to jail crowding, most arrestees with any kind of stable past go home to wait for arraignment and trial. And yet, we want to believe that most people, even criminals, are very much like us. This group is, which is why it is rare for them to commit crimes.

The entire criminal justice system is based on what should happen to people like this who commit crimes. It works for this small percentage.

Hustlers. By far the biggest population in jails today, hustlers are low-level street criminals: drug users, pushers, thieves, prostitutes, and robbers. Almost all are addicted to one or more drugs or just take any drugs that they can find, buy, or steal. Most gangbangers fall into this category, no matter how much they try to romanticize their image.

It is a subculture and a way of life. In the early 1980s as part of a sociology project, I spent a short time "being homeless": living in shelters, eating at missions, and hustling. While Ronald Reagan was on TV saying that the homeless chose to be homeless, I was hearing the same thing from their lips.

I was told that any obligation—job, mortgage payment, or family—was a form of slavery. That only the homeless were truly free. That it was stupid to work when others were willing to and would give you money for the asking. There was no distinction between charities, panhandling, and government aid—the smart were given money, the stupid gave it.

There are many, many details that I could give you about this stratum of society. That would be a book in itself, and I recommend *Beggars and Thieves* by Mark S. Fleisher. In broad strokes, life is largely based around drugs and money for drugs. People who have never dealt with it often underestimate the power of addiction. Some addicts will and have killed, prostituted themselves and their children, betrayed family members, and sold children for enough drugs to get through the day.

Violence is common with this group for very logical reasons. They will fight to defend their territory and possessions because there is no other authority that will do so. They will use violence to secure drugs or money to get drugs. They will fight for reputation because a victim reputation will ensure future victimization. Most of the time, the violence is against other hustlers.

Citizens do not frequent the same places as hustlers. When they do, they are often healthier and stronger than the hustler...and the hustler finds guilt, intimidation, and smell to be as effective as violence, in most cases with far less risk.

My first use of force in the jail was interesting. I was challenged by a gangbanger and it was going to go physical. I had studied martial arts for ten years at the time and had only a handful of real encounters bouncing in a casino. This was different—a vicious gangbanger killer criminal in a venue with no rules and no help... basically a lot of bullshit went through my mind. I forced myself to grab him.

It felt like he was made out of cheese. I'd been playing with college level athletes for ten years. This was an undernourished, drug-addicted punk. In my own mind, I'd created this vicious image but it wasn't real. What would have happened if I had responded to the image, to the fear instead of duty? Career would have been much shorter and less pleasant, that's for sure.

When a hustler goes to violence, it will follow the dynamics mentioned previously. They will Monkey Dance, less for status with a citizen than for territory. The groups are prone to the GMD. Once a hustler starts relying on predation, the dynamic changes. See below.

They will be likely to use a weapon. Most carry a weapon of

The Continuum of Evil

Actor's Motivation	Victim's Area of Loss
whim	*whim*
social status	*social status*
social identity	*social identity*
physical security	*physical security*
survival	*survival*

If motivation and loss are at equal levels on the chart, the act is usually justifiable. If the angle is descending from left to right, the act is evil. Ascending, good.

The Continuum of Evil is my contribution to an essentially useless but interesting ways of looking at things. Abraham Maslow described the famous Maslow's Hierarchy of Needs. He pointed out that biology—food, water, and not being eaten—always came first. Only after you had food and weren't in immediate peril did you start to worry about "safety needs," the basic security that you will have food and water tomorrow as well. When that was assured, you would look for love, affection, and a social system to fit into.

Once you had a social system, you would start looking for secure status within that group and within yourself, self-esteem, and the esteem of your peers. Only when that was satisfied would you look to a higher calling and be unafraid to walk your own path in life.

With respectful apology to Dr. Maslow, I'm cribbing his hierarchy, applying it to two people and rephrasing "self-actualization" as "whims" to construct a way to measure evil, and to simplify the language.

> ## The Continuum of Evil *(continued)*
> Breaking it down, you have: survival, physical security, social identity, social status, and whim.
>
> Generally, society sees aggressive interactions at the same level as excusable, justified, or right, and interactions at a low level for a higher justification as wrong. It is okay to kill someone (attacking them at the survival need level) to save your own life, but not so that you will have food tomorrow. It is bad to kill someone because he insulted your family, nation, or team, but worse to kill for status in your gang. Killing on a whim is the worst of all.
>
> Theft is often attacking at the physical security level. Stealing food, a physical security attack with a survival motive, is easily excused. Stealing food from someone who is also hungry is less so.
>
> It works the other way, too. Dying in an attempt to save yourself is just dying. Dying to save your family (who are as much physical security as social) is commendable. Dying to save your tribe or platoon is heroic. Dying to prove your status in the group is considered a sure gateway to sainthood in the cultures that condone the act—stupidity, or brainwashing to outsiders. Dying for an ideal or a whim is martyrdom, something very important and powerful to insiders, inexplicable and fanatical to outsiders.
>
> *Caveat:* This is just an interesting way to try to quantify the unquantifiable. It is not important.

some kind—often a knife—but I've also seen a welding hammer and a rock in a sock. They do not fear jail in any way and their sense of right and wrong is grossly distorted—without regret, remorse, or hesitation, they will use more force than a citizen would consider.

Jail is a pit stop for this lifestyle. It is literally a necessary part of the life cycle. Fleisher made statements in his book that I checked later with the criminals in my custody. One of his statements was that hustlers rarely if ever are arrested and go to jail unless they want to. When they feel sick, extremely hungry, or cold, they will arrange to be seen doing a minor crime or picked up on a warrant sweep. In jail, they are cleaned up, given food and medical care and generally made healthy enough to continue their lifestyle. The choice to go to jail is a balancing act between wants, such as food, and fear of withdrawals.

Needless to say, jail is neither a deterrent nor rehabilitative for these criminals. It is literally R&R for their lifestyle. It is enabling.

Drugs have long-term effects on the addicts. As attackers, they tend to be slow, clumsy, and stupid. Not necessarily slower than you expect. They can fall into the flurry attack of a killing rage very easily, but the brain and body damage show.

When I first started, one of our inmates was a lightweight boxer working his way into the pros. He was fairly intelligent, in great shape, and ugly to fight—and just starting his crack habit. The last time I saw him he was toothless, could barely remember his own name, and had lost a leg to infection.

Predators. Predators see you as a resource. If they attack, it will be from the greatest advantage they can muster. We've described the dynamic already. Predators range from the hustler who has found a relatively safe and efficient way to get what he or she wants to the true psychopath to the serial killer/rapist.

Hustlers will get money for drugs, frequently through robbery. Rather than use direct violence, many can convince a victim to "donate" money with mere intimidation—standing too close with some friends nearby or showing a weapon. Occasionally, one will learn that a quick application of violence can get the desired result quickly and with less fuss than intimidation.

There is a video on the Internet of a Russian crack addict walking up to a fifteen-year-old girl, throwing her to the ground and stomping on her head many times before going through her purse. He then stands and stomps on her head some more before going through her pockets. When I show this to students I have to emphasize that this is not some superpredator. This is a skinny crackhead who has found a quick, safe, and easy way to get a purse. It is brutal. It is not unusual.

Sociopath is really a sliding scale and a label. People are people, and my pain is more important to me than your pain. My family's pain is more important to me than yours. 9/11 affected me more than the much more numerous and horrible deaths in Bosnia. As you move along the continuum of evil, the Narcissistic Personality Disorder feels that he is far more important than you; the true sociopath doesn't acknowledge your reality at all.

As a side effect, Hollywood aside, most sociopaths aren't that bright. They can be charming. They can be well spoken. They stick to what they know. The big flaw in their reasoning is that by not accepting that other people are really "real," they have a difficult time learning from other people's mistakes.

All predators will be somewhere on the antisocial spectrum. They have decided that what they want is more important than what you have or are.

The serial predator is a process predator for whom the *act* is all-important. I've known several and can only tell you that outside of the crimes, they sometimes seemed very normal. One was a creepy weird old dude. One was a blue-collar regular joe. One was a hard drinking good-ol'-boy rancher. One was an articulate young man. Another was very intelligent and seemed normal, provided you didn't see his artwork.

Detectives interviewed an inmate in our custody for murder. They passed on to us as a safety briefing that the inmate had said that stabbing his victim was the biggest rush, the most awesome feeling of power, and the greatest experience of his life. He stated that from the time of the stabbing he had been obsessed with finding an opportunity to do it again without getting caught.*

For most true predators, jail is meaningless. It just gives them a different victim pool. For the hustler who has learned to prey, his predation is very dependent on his quality of victim. He can usually safely intimidate and rob a law-abiding citizen. In jail, retaliation from his potential victims or action from the guards increase the risk, so most quickly revert to hustler status inside the jail, scamming.

---

* Criminals lie all the time, especially to officers. I'll report what was said but do not assume it was truth. Many professional investigators have published influential works in which they were clearly snowed. FYI.

Special Circumstances: Mentally Ill and Drugs in the System.
The inmate was kicking the door, screaming and yelling threats in a
separation cell after being booked. These days, we would have just
let him scream and kick until he got tired, but in the Old Days™ we
went into the cell and dealt with it. I stood at the window as he was
screaming, "Come on in! Let's die together!!!" He was laughing. I've
done this enough that I have a system. Someone else slips the key in
the door, silently turns it and whips the door open while the threat
is talking. I enter while his mind is trying to shift from talking to
fighting, spin him by his elbow and use the concrete bench to trip
him off his feet and get him face down.

This guy heard the lock turn. He was ready when I entered. I
closed past the fists, turned the elbow and pushed, and he leapt onto
the bench. He was insanely fast. I stayed with him, not wanting to
give him the space to strike, and jumped onto the bench next to him.
He started to turn and I swept his legs out, spinning him in the air
at almost shoulder height. For one second, time was frozen and he
was falling head first toward the concrete floor. I imagined a head-
line "Corrections Martial Artist Kills Poor, Misunderstood, Mental
Patient" when my backup materialized and caught him in midair.
Cuffs went on his legs and ankles.

I saw him a couple of days later and I was surprised. He was
lucid, calm. Not psychotic at all. He told me the PCP had worn off.
PCP. I'd heard that people under the influence could be insanely
strong. I didn't know about the speed.

Mental illness and drugs can mimic each other in a fight. In
essence, parts of your brain go offline. The part that says "this is
a bad idea" or "that hurts," for instance. We had an inmate try to
gouge out his own eyes with his thumbs. He got one.

I can break the differences down into motivation and stops.

The unpredictability of the mentally ill is extremely challenging.
One of the very few times I have been successfully sucker-punched
was by a very elderly schizophrenic lady. We were talking. She hit
me and just kept on talking. There were no pre-assault cues, no telegraphs...other than the hand lashing out, there was no indication in
her face or body that she was even striking.

Dealing with sane and sober people, we assume that they do things for reasons. A schizophrenic or someone on hallucinogens may not be seeing the same world that you are. He or she may literally be responding to a cue that is invisible to you but real to them. It makes them hard to predict.

Stops are the point when a normal person would quit or would choose not to engage. Outnumbered or presence of officers would prevent most people from starting a situation. A mentally ill person may not notice these conditions.

Pain, injury, or exhaustion will often stop a normal person. Again, the mentally ill may not notice or may ignore these stops. They may even respond further into the survival reflex and pour on more speed and power.

Deputy Leader reminded me of an inmate she fought long ago. He had attempted to hang himself and when deputies responded, he was blue. They cut him down and he began to fight. The deputies used numbers and force to get handcuffs and leg irons on and the inmate still fought for over thirty minutes with a series of officers. At one point after he was restrained, he threw an officer off so hard that she permanently injured her back.

"Excited Delirium" is a catch-all term for what may be a complex disorder that manifests in different situations. That's a fancy way to say that we don't know what causes it. The threats in this condition are usually but not always long-term stimulant abusers (cocaine, meth, PCP), sometimes (but not always) on the drug at the time (and not always a particularly high dose), sometimes (but not always) have a history of mental illness, and sometimes (but not always) all of the above.

They appear the same way, though: incoherent and screaming, violent and aggressive, often naked because the body temperature shoots up (a liver temperature of 108 degrees has been recorded), incredibly strong and fast, impervious to pain and, for some reason, they tend to break glass when they see it. This is the nightmare opponent. A person in this state will continue to fight long after exhaustion and will often fight against a group of officers.

Physiology and physics still work—with enough mass and leverage they can be controlled. Shutting down the brain (through damage or strangulation) still works. When finally restrained, they are at great risk for just suddenly dying. A fight with officers may be the most stressful and exhausting event of the threat's life, combined with some cocktail of drugs and brain chemicals that pushes them beyond the normal limits of endurance; and pain added to a heart weakened by stimulant addiction results, sometimes, in sudden death after the fight is over.

section 4.3: rationalizations

One of the things that has always amazed me about criminals is the mental gymnastics they do to convince themselves that they are both the good guys and the victims. I know that everyone feels that they are the heroes of their own private stories, but deep down, I always thought there were some limits of depravity that couldn't be rationalized. So far, I'm wrong.

On the same day, I've had one arrestee say, "I'm not a real criminal; I just steal stuff. I don't hurt nobody." And another say, "So I beat the shit out of that guy, but I'm not a criminal. I never stole anything."

Two inmates got in a fight in a cell. It turns out they were betting on cards, betting blowjobs. Both considered the other gay, but felt that they were "real men."

One inmate is incarcerated for stabbing an eight-year-old girl to death. The little girl was a hero: She died jumping between her father and the man trying to stab him. It doesn't bother the killer's conscience at all. He says he is confident he will get manslaughter "at the most." Since the girl wasn't the person he intended to kill, he feels it wasn't murder.

"Sarge, do you think I'm a criminal?" an inmate asked me.

"Dunno, what'd you do?"

"I beat my father with a baseball bat. I cracked his skull."

"Yeah, you're a criminal."

"Oh. Am I a bad person?"

"Good people don't beat people with baseball bats."

"Oh." What was he thinking? Was he hoping I'd say, "Hell, son, you're a fine human being. Lots of good people beat other people with bats every day."?

One more, and I'll move on. Early in my career, an inmate was reluctantly talking about his crime. "It wasn't *me*, Miller. It's not like me. It was the cocaine. I'd never do a thing like that if it wasn't for the coke." How much cocaine would you have to snort before you would break into a house and rape and sodomize an eighty-year-old woman? There isn't enough cocaine in the world for most criminals. The drugs don't do the crimes.

Rationalization is the internal process of convincing oneself that the violent horrible thing you want to do is honorable, logical, and justified. For the most part, from the perspective of self-defense, rationalization is rarely relevant. It happens entirely in the attacker's head and you must deal with the physical reality of the assault more than the threat's mindset. For the stalker or the predator, you will know nothing of what goes on in his head until the attack. For the Monkey Dance, it is largely mutual. For the process predator, it is internal. For the predator intent on robbery, does it make any difference to you if he tells himself he needs drugs or if he tells himself he's striking a blow against an oppressive society?

Often, there is an interview stage in an assault, a moment when the threat sizes up the potential victim's alertness, confidence, and willingness to engage. If the focus of the assault is on gaining something, the meekest victim is chosen.

Sometimes the interview is used to attempt to rationalize or provoke a Monkey Dance or to set up a pretext for a more violent ego-based attack. Especially after a blow to self-esteem, a threat will start looking for an excuse to do damage. He will try to get you to say or do something to justify his actions.

There is a skill to avoiding this. I call it "not giving away hooks." It is very much like the Big Dog tactic discussed in the section on the Monkey Dance. Stay rational and calm; treat the statements, no matter how provocative, as thoughtful questions. There is a limit to this, though. At a certain point too much reasonableness can be interpreted by the threat as manipulation, and he has his justification to strike. If I feel it getting to that point, my usual defense is to call the threat on it.

I can't honestly say I remember this next conversation. I have a conversation like this about twice a week. Daily, when I'm working maximum security.

"This is bullshit, Sarge, and you know it!" The inmate is angry, trying to work himself into a righteous rage and put on a show for the other inmates. He is also trying to get me to say something either in anger or dismissive that he can use as a pretext to escalate or for further proof in his own mind that he is the victim, oppressed by the forces of society. Something as little as "Shut up!" is enough to give him what he wants.

So I say, "Take a deep breath. You're going to the hole. There's nothing you can say right now that will make it better." I keep my voice calm. Rate, tone, pitch, and volume are all low and slow.

"Fuck that! That guard's a punk! If I saw him on the street..." The inmate starts using hot button words and threats to either provoke me into action OR to see if I will be weak and let him go on with his rant—more points in status from the other inmates. This is the point where I have to call him on it and shut it down.

So I shut it down, staying calm. "Let it go. You don't need more paper and that sounded like the start of a threat."

"Fuck that! Fuck your threat and fuck you!" Line crossed.

I like using names and standing close when I'm shutting someone down physically or verbally. "Mr. XXX, do you want to make this personal?" He freezes for a second, so I continue, "I'm trying really hard to keep you from doing something stupid and you aren't listening, so I'm going to ask: Do you want to make this personal with me?"

"No, man. I'm sorry, Sarge. I was just pissed off."

"That's okay. Don't say anything else right now."

First thing—as you've noticed—the majority of my examples will be from jail. I work in a jail. Most of the conflicts I have are with criminals. I have a huge advantage in that they know me, and I know them. Reputation is huge. I really don't get into a lot of conflicts outside of work.

In jail or out of jail, in this type of scenario, asking if it's personal does two things. It raises the stakes. Monkey Dancing is not really personal. It's about rungs on the ladder, not who sits on the rungs. Except for the process predator, predation is about the money (or whatever), not the specific person. Violence usually involves damage. When it's personal, it's *about* damage. Punishment. Punishment is worse.

Second, by asking it as a question, it forces the threat to abandon the idea of getting me to give him a hook. From that point, if the threat escalates, he no longer has the illusion that the attack is honorable or logical or justified. Most people who are on this fence need the rationalization, because they want to believe that they are the good guys.

Violence in the past is the strongest indicator of violence in the future: Predators rarely cease to prey. If you have the sense to avoid places where violence happens, you should have the sense to avoid violent people. Most people choose to be blind to the failings of people they care about. You can't afford to be. If someone is a violent criminal, he is a violent criminal even if he is the father of your children. He will continue to hurt people.

There are also people who may not seem violent themselves, but violence and chaos seem to follow them around. Consciously or unconsciously, some people manipulate the people around them to increase the drama for their own excitement. It results in violence too often. I once heard, "That man could start a brawl at a Quaker Peace Rally." Someone like that will get you involved in unnecessary danger. Leave him alone.

Violence in the past is the strongest indicator of violence in the future. This is also true for victims. Not only do sons of abusive fathers tend to grow up into abusers but also many daughters spend their lives bouncing from one abusive relationship to another. Early childhood modeling imprints what a relationship is supposed to be, right or wrong. Somehow, molesters who prey on children can tell if a child has been abused in the past and know that a child who has once been a victim is very likely to be an easy victim again. This pattern is subconscious and pernicious. If you have been a victim of violent or sexual crimes multiple times, please see a counselor. If you seem to go from bad relationship to bad relationship, see a counselor.

section 4.4: what makes a violent predator?

Does it matter? In the moment of violence, you must deal with what is happening; the past does not matter. If someone is trying to cut your throat, the threat's motives or mindset or reasons or excuses are irrelevant. Those are things for his defense attorney to trot out in an attempt to mitigate his deeds.

Yet, the subject is interesting and worth theorizing.

There are theories. Lots of them. Most are crap. Lonnie Athens' "violentization" process as outlined in Richard Rhodes' book, *Why They Kill,* fits my experience best in that it explains why not all children brought up the same way become violent. Simply, the ones that become violent adults were the ones that violence worked for. If a child or young adult attempts to bully or lash out and is rewarded (*see* "Operant Conditioning," Section 5.4) by the positive reinforcement of approval or the negative reward of their tormenter backing off, they will continue to be violent. If escalating violence works, they will escalate.

One of my favorite, and in my opinion, most insightful explorers into what makes a violent preditor is Stanton Samenow in *Inside the Criminal Mind.* It is chilling when he points out that some children may provoke their own abuse by refusing to acknowledge any level of punishment. Most of us discipline our children with a word, a stern look, or by withholding a privilege. This works, however, because the child lets it work. We want the child to quit throwing the ball in the house, so we tell them. If they know it is wrong, they get the "Trouble" look. If that doesn't work, we escalate to the raised voice with the full name. If that doesn't work, send the kid to his room...but if you think about it, this process of escalation continues until the child starts to comply. Samenow avers that a very small percentage of children do not choose to comply no matter how far the punishment escalates, even into vicious abuse. The parents in these cases did not begin as abusive and did not abuse their other children, if they had any. It is very uncomfortable to think that even in a very small percentage of cases, victims of child abuse create the situation.

To clarify, this does not justify abuse and if you read this and think, "Oh, it's okay I hit my kid, then. Little shit had it comin'," then I'd like to politely tell you that you are full of shit and need to burn in hell.

Where Samenow shines is in describing the adult accomplished criminal. No matter how it arises, the predator, once created, remains a predator. No system of rehabilitation has been able to change this basic personality trait.

The Criminal Personality

Whether it is inborn or a product of environment, there is a criminal personality. Actually, there are a handful with different flavors and quirks, but with a single factor that makes them behave in a criminal fashion: They consider themselves more important than their victims and their desires more important than the rules that allow people to live in a society. Whether the behavior is driven by a Narcissistic Personality Disorder, in which case the self-esteem is so great that the criminal feels he deserves and should have anything he wants or the Antisocial Personality Disorder in which other people are without value—just toys, tools, or resources— the behavior gets to the same place. Use and abuse of other humans.

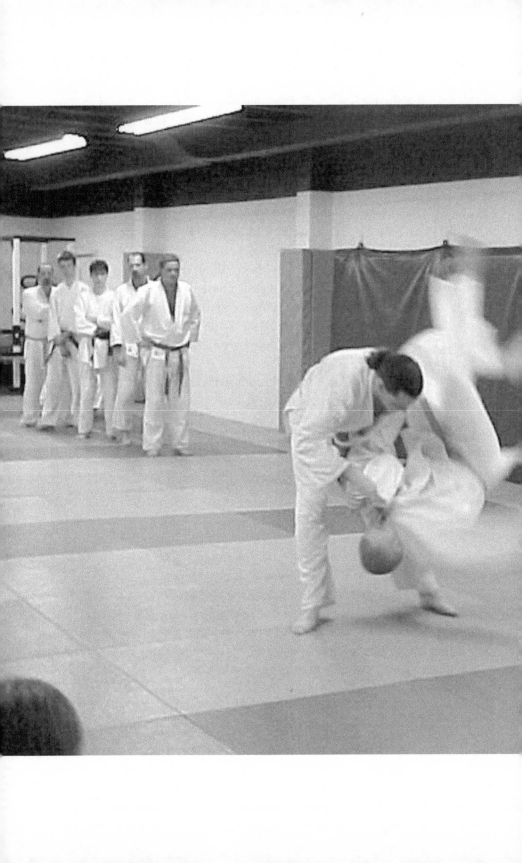

CHAPTER 5: TRAINING

section 5.1: the flaw in the drill

In the end, a martial artist is training to injure, cripple, or kill another human being. In any drill where students are not regularly hospitalized, there is a DELIBERATE flaw, a deliberate break from the needs of reality introduced in the name of safety. In every drill you teach, you must consciously know what the flaw is and make your students aware of it.

Let me be clear. There is no way to exactly replicate breaking people without breaking them, and a large part of the history of the martial arts has been in finding safe ways to approximate that action. Tony Blauer calls it the search for "the best fake stuff out there." Bryan, a friend and Jujutsu student, but also a former competitive fencer, pointed out that by making the weapons safe, fencing was able to maintain the majority of its lethal technique (though the sport has changed vastly in response to technological development). In unarmed combatives, with no weapon to "make safe," the techniques themselves had to be altered. Unless the students and teachers are very aware, this alteration becomes the "right" way to do the technique.

Generally, there are three ways that something can be a flaw:

(1) When the drill sets an unrealistic expectation of what an attack will be like—too far, too slow, from the front, too light (violates the Four Basic Truths of Section 3.2).

(2) When the drill allows techniques that would be unsafe or crippling for the person using them in real life: boxing gloves or nice warmed-up high kicks, for instance.

(3) Most damning, when the solution to the drill is based on the FLAW: using medium speed defenses to defeat slow-motion attacks; blocking; or the bad kind of flow (teacher leading student), mentioned later in the chapter.

Since effectiveness of a technique is based on targeting, timing,

Throw line
Courtesy Chris Luttrell

and power generation, many flaws attempts to alter or omit one of these three aspects.

Let's look at some common flaws and where these flaws provide safety and where and when they get mistaken for good fighting tactics.

Flaws in static drills. Static drills are repetitive actions, usually simple techniques. When used without a partner, such as line drills, hitting the heavy bag, or Karate *kata*, they do not require safety modification and so can be very good training. Properly used they allow the student to practice excellent power generation and body mechanics without fear of injury.

The flaws in static drills are in what is absent. It is hard to develop targeting by punching air. The subtle pressure and dynamics of moving an opponent or breaking his balance are integral to making grappling, takedowns, and locks work and can't be practiced without a partner. This is one of the main reasons that solo *kata*, shadow boxing, and line drills are disparaged in grappling schools: It's a bad way to train for grappling.

Also missing are the intricacies of targeting on a moving opponent and the skill to adapt to the situation as it changes. Memorized combinations applied in air almost never work the same way on a body that reacts and resists. The feeling of impact (even when you hit someone, it can hurt you) and the feeling of being hit are also missing, which can lead to freezing in a real conflict when it doesn't feel like you expected.

Properly trained, static drills can be very good tools for picking up the skills of violence. By removing the opponent, you can strike with full power, speed, intent, and savagery. These drills, unlike others, do not create bad habits, provided the instructor knows what he is teaching. Properly trained, the student can perform any action correctly—but the absence of chaos during practice often leads to the student freezing when presented with chaos.

There are two more negative affects that relying on static drills can bring to your training. The first is that because there is no opponent, and often in older styles no consistent explanation of the dynamics, generations of instructors (with no realistic idea of combat) have imagined what the invisible opponent is doing, and those imaginings tend to be tied closer to movies than to reality. These imaginings build on themselves over time. For an example, there is a basic Karate technique in which the fist is held high at the same-side ear and brought down to the centerline, fist in front of the nose, elbow down (I learned it as the "inside block" since it moves to the inside. Other styles call it an outside block, since it comes from the outside). This is usually taught as a block, used on an imaginary opponent at polite dueling distance. The exact same technique, according to Champ Thomas in *Boxing's Dirty Tricks and Outlaw Killer Punches* when practiced at very close range is illegal in boxing due to a number of deaths in the early twentieth century.

The second negative possibility is that given a technique or set of techniques that was designed by someone who knew about violence and staying alive, people seem almost driven to mess with them. Things are added or changed to bring them into line with what the instructor imagines a fight looks like. There is a style of Okinawan Karate that I admire very much that originally had no closed-fist strikes in the system. This made sense to me—an open-handed strike can do as much or more damage than a fist with less risk of injury to you. It was one of the clues to me that this was a true fighting system. Later, they added closed-fist strikes to bring them in line with what other styles were doing in competition.

Flaws in active cooperative drills. I define active drills as those that involve two or more students but where the students' actions are scripted and/or the goal is not to win in any way. Examples would be partner line drills, *uchikomi* drills in Judo or *siniwalli* drills in Arnis, and flow drills.

Flow can mean many things to me, depending on the context and my mood. Sometimes it is a serious flaw that can pervade an entire system and sometimes it is common sense. When it means moving with the natural lines of force of your own body (e.g., not throwing your right hip and left fist forward), no problem.

When used as "reading and exploiting the rhythm of the opponents movement," it is a dueling or sparring artifact that is suicidal in a sudden assault. Flow as rhythm involves time, and time is precious in a sudden assault. In a duel or a sparring match where you start at a safe distance and slowly work to your damage distance, there can be many "probing" attacks to get to know your opponent and exploit his preferences in timing and personal rhythm. It takes a minimum of three beats for a human to extrapolate the simplest rhythm. In combat, each of those beats is an attempt to injure you. The concept of using rhythm to defend in an ambush is deciding to take three potentially lethal hits so that you can devise a more elegant response.

When it means transitioning from technique to technique seamlessly (i.e., in a lock flow drill), it is pretty and impressive but sometimes stupid. Especially with locks and immobilizations, you only transition from bad techniques to good ones. You never transition for the sake of the transition. If the first technique is good, you don't give it away for something that might go bad. That's different for striking, where each technique is a small explosive slice of time, but you get the idea.

Sometimes "flow" is used to describe what is essentially a sensitivity drill, such as sticky hands. You can learn things from it, but when it is used (and this is almost always subconscious) by the instructor to lead his students to move in a certain way so that his techniques will work, it is horrible and dangerous.

In any cooperative drill, you have a real target so you must have a safety flaw.

Targeting is one of the most common things to derail to make a drill safe. In many styles, punches are pulled so that there is no contact. In some drills, such as *siniwalli*, the students strike at each other's weapon and beginners stay out of range to prevent accidental contact. These students are literally being taught to miss, practicing misses to the tune of a hundred or a thousand misses a class. People do pull punches in real encounters. When Bryan was grabbed from behind, he spun and fired three fast punches into the threat's chest, punches so fast and perfectly controlled that they made loud snapping noises against the threat's jacket and did no damage whatsoever. Bryan did exactly what he had trained to do.

Power generation and power transmission are sometimes degraded in cooperative drills but they rarely need to be. The same attention can be paid to proper structure and lines of movement as can be in solo drills.

Timing is the flaw that I personally incorporate the most often. I believe that going in slow motion will be physically impossible in most real encounters so I have little fear of creating a bad habit on that score. Where it becomes a bad habit is when students either cheat on the drill, speeding up to make a technique work, or when they practice doing things that they can only do because of the speed of the drill, such as blocking baseball bats with their forearms or snatching punches out of the air. There are other timing flaws, such as the "my turn/your turn," which might get students to pause in a real situation.

Scripting, where students practice a specific defense to a specific attack can have many of the missing elements of the static drills. In addition, if the attacks and the responses are not realistic—such as the *uke* with an openly displayed knife lunging from far out of range so that *tori* can catch the wrist and neatly lock him up—the habits created will be useless and the students may freeze because a real encounter is so different from what they were taught to expect.

Meta-flaws in dynamic (competitive) drills. Dynamic drills involve maximum freedom of movement and choice in a training environment. This is sparring or *randori* or *kumite*. Rollin' and brawlin'. Within the rules, you can do anything you can think of in an attempt to win.

There are meta-flaws in sparring that have to be well understood by the instructor. Because they are dynamic and because we know that fights are dynamic, there is a tendency to use sparring as a reality check. Since most people have learned about physical conflict by watching entertaining shows (whether professional sports, movies, or "reality TV," it is *entertainment*), or from class, and since sparring looks more like this image than, say, basics or line drills, they intuitively believe it is more "real." It isn't. A real fight for your life is NOTHING like sparring.

Even more important in the meta-flaws is that sparring is fun and active—so habits gained in sparring are deeper and more durable than in less engaging practice. It also looks more like what a student expects a fight to look like than other training methods, which reinforces assumptions derived from entertainment.

Almost twenty-five years ago, I asked my Karate *sensei* why we practiced *kihon* (basics) and *kata* when the techniques we used in sparring looked nothing like *kata*. He didn't have a good answer, just some vague nonsense about discipline and muscle development. Twenty years ago, after my first ugly brawl in the casino, I remember sucking wind, shaking, and thinking, "Shit, that wasn't *anything* like sparring."

Most martial artists will never have that big ugly brawl and they are perfectly free to believe that sparring is as close as it gets to real life. Sparring is worthwhile anyway if only because it is fun.

Flaws in dynamic drills. Just as power, timing, and targeting are integral to fighting, one or more of these must be screwed up in order to practice safely.

Light contact or non-contact sparring (pulling punches) degrades both power generation and targeting. It is easy to degenerate into a game of tag where ineffective speed is rewarded. It is much, much easier to hit an opponent with a flick of extended fingers with all your weight on your toes than it is to land a solid blow that might disable. If they are considered equal as far as points, the players will go for the easier one. It becomes a habit.

Pulling punches is literally practicing to miss. Targeting is screwed up by forbidding targets (e.g., no striking below the belt; no strikes to the face) or over-generalizing targets. If someone trains to hit "the body," they lose the effect of striking specifically for the floating ribs, the liver, the solar plexus, the bladder, etc. By practicing imprecision they never develop precision. Same for the head. Most of the head is more damaging to your hand than to the person you hit.

There is also tournament targeting that was designed for safety but quickly became the "right way" to do the technique. The Muay Thai round kick to the lower quads has a well-deserved reputation for power and effect, but drop the same technique about three inches and it is crippling. Outside of sport, it is important to practice the crippling techniques.

Timing can become very sophisticated in sparring, which is a flaw in and of itself. People do not attack with a knife the same way that they spar with one. It is fast, close, and staccato. Sparring is often a chess match of distance and timing. Assault is an overwhelming onslaught. The skills don't transfer.

I often use slow motion as my flaw in active drills for the reasons mentioned before: I don't believe it can become a habit. However, it is easy for students to cheat by speeding up with a slow opponent or doing things that they couldn't do at speed, such as snatch the end of a baton out of the air.

Safety equipment can create bad training habits, also. Striking with an unprotected fist is hard. Extremely skilled boxers tend to break their hands in street altercations. Gloves also throw off your distancing. Armor is better, in my opinion, but it still can't protect joints and a good blow to the head can still damage the neck, even in heavy armor.

A gloved fist doesn't cause damage in quite the same way as a naked strike, either. It turns the punch into a push where most of the damage comes from the brain bouncing against the inside of the skull. Unprotected hands, used properly, tend to fracture the bones of the skull around the eye, or the cheekbone, or the jaw.

Most styles start much too far away to simulate a sudden assault. Either they are working from the "dueling assumption" or the drill was introduced to substitute distance for time—by making the attacker reach, it gave the defender a little more time to work on the subtleties of the defense. Poor distancing can become a serious flaw in many ways. Entire classes of techniques can arise to fit a situation that only exists in training (blocks); timing will be off. Power generation for damage will be off.

section 5.2: kata as a training exercise

First, there are two distinct types of *kata* in the Japanese tradition. Most martial arts are familiar with the solo *kata* of Karate. In these *kata*, the *karateka* goes through a series of predetermined moves. Two-man *kata* are common in the older styles of Japanese martial arts. In these, two practitioners act on each other in a scripted fashion. I've already described some of the inherent flaws in scripted drills, but these training methods did not survive for hundreds of years because they sucked. Here, I want to point out some of the advantages.

Solo Kata. Understand that I have only dabbled in Karate, though my wife is a practitioner.

Occasionally, I would have an encounter, often an intense one, and later see the action in my wife's Karate *kata*. One time, I was the only officer on the booking floor on a night shift. I heard a sound coming from one of our group holding rooms and I slid the window cover open. I saw one fresh arrestee slamming kicks into another who was laying on the ground.

I called for back-up and keyed the door open. Procedure would have been to wait for back-up but in my estimation, the kid on the ground was about to be kicked to death. I reached in, grabbed the kicker by the hood, yanked him out of the room, and slammed him against the wall outside. I applied cuffs without a problem; he was stunned by the speed. When I started doing the report, I found out that he had been a state champion wrestler a few years before.

The body mechanics looked like a basic *kata*. The reach and grab looked like a lunge punch. In the *kata,* this is followed by a ninety-degree turn and an outside block with the punching hand. I had his hood in that hand, so it pulled him off-balance, forward, head almost to my hip, and spun him up to face away from me. The next move in *kata* is a reverse punch with the other hand. In real life, my palm slammed and pinned him against the wall.

It was effective. The body mechanics were identical to *kata*. Not a single move was the way any Karate instructor had ever explained it to me.

I am not saying that *kata* is the optimal or even a good way to train. What I am saying is that from my experience, the mechanics of Karate *kata* are extremely functional in real life.

To me, it looks like *kata* is all about hands, shoulders, and hips working together simultaneously with a drop in center of gravity (COG). This is one of the most potent systems of power generation. This is a potent system regardless of whether the action is interpreted as a strike, a lock, or a throw.

The more possibilities you see in anything, the more options you have. Since the actions can be interpreted effectively in so many ways, *kata* may be more powerful as a training tool if you see none of those (or all of them) than if you decide it is just one of them. As long as the hips, hands, shoulders, and COG work together, there is no difference anyway. *Karateka* get in their own way when they try to dig into the "deeper secrets" of their movement. Learn to move. *Kata* is excellent for that. Then reproduce or experience the dynamics of actual conflict and you will see how much really valid technique there is in the old forms.

Two-Man *Kata*.

> "Kata *is to be done in an air of distrust.*"
> —Shuzuk Shitama, 16th *dai-shihan* of Sosuishitsu-ryu

Not everyone does *kata* the same way and not everyone will get the same things out of it that I did. I know people with teaching certificates in my style who cannot fight and I know some who are devastating but did not follow this training path. This is what *I* got out of *kata*.

The two-man *kata* of traditional Japanese Jujutsu were a very sophisticated training method. You were teaching young *bushi* to kill an armed and armored warrior quickly. Training armor wouldn't help, since you were training to defeat real armor. If you altered the technique for safety, the alteration would become a habit and the warrior would pull his punches under stress. The solution was for *uke* to attack with full power, speed, and commitment. *Tori* countered, also, with full power, speed, and commitment and then *uke* would do the one specific thing that would be counter-intuitive on the battlefield but would save him in *kata*. In the Sosuishi-ryu *kata, Tori ire, uke* drops his sword to prevent falling on the *tsuba,* with full body weight focused over his floating ribs. In *Kawashime, uke* goes limp to prevent his spine from shearing. In *Munadori, uke* must jump with toe flexion or his collarbone is shattered. Et cetera.

Kata can be done many ways. Most learn the forms and learn them well enough to teach and move on. They become stale, stylistic rituals.

But there is more here. Not from all instructors and not for all students, but there is much more. When Bo and I were training *kata* to prepare for our certification, it was very intense. It started with learning the moves and then speeding them up. Then *sensei* insisted we add true commitment. When we were *uke*, we struck at each other (with *boken* to the head) full force, full power. The only thing in *uke*'s mind was "to cut." If I hand someone a *boken* and tell them to hit me in the head as hard as they can, very, very few will even be able to do it in a half-hearted way. Most that do swing, when I look in their eyes, will freeze at the last minute, sometimes even pulling muscles to stop from hitting. From that point on, Bo and I trusted each other to strike to kill, for real, every time.

Then *sensei* insisted we "wait in stillness" before moving (to be fair, we'd always done this, but with the introduction of killing intent there was a new level and new consequences). This changed the drill. If *uke* sensed any movement from *tori, uke* altered the attack. In other words, *uke* would strike at the head and if *tori* moved too soon *uke* would drop the strike and slam you in the ribs. *Tori* learned to wait and then explode.

Tachypsychia is the term for the sensation that everything is going in slow motion. It sometimes happens under extreme stress. This is the only training I've ever undergone or even heard of that taught you to consciously access this state.

The last stage was to apply this without the safety of *kata*. In other words, we would assume starting position and *uke* could attack in any way that he chose. Freeform *kata*, if you will. We found that the responses were rarely out of *kata*, but highlighted the principles.

What did we get from this? Some criminal screaming that he's going to kill me just isn't intimidating anymore. There is more time in a second than I need. I can be still and I can explode. I learned to deal with what is there and not what I expected.

What did it cost? It was dangerous. One of my *ukes* tried to do an intuitive breakfall and his collarbone shattered into three pieces. I sprained my neck several times going limp a fraction of a second late. I still remember that second of slow-motion time when I realized that Bo was about to land on his bent neck with full force and me yanking to get his body over in the last six inches of falling space... spraining his neck badly but not killing him.

And there was a cool-down period. For much of the last part of this training, I couldn't spar. I was on a hair-trigger and couldn't even think of a non-lethal response to anything. It took a while to wear off, because even in a maximum security jail that level of preparation is frowned upon by society.

section 5.3: responses to the four basic truths

Section 3.2 was about the four aspects of a sudden assault that are hardest to train for and most unfamiliar to martial artists. To recap, assaults happen *fast, hard, close,* and with *surprise.*

There are specific ways to train to deal with these truths about assault. Most importantly, the very concept of "fairness" has no place in the discussion of predatory assault. The victim can't afford to be fair, and the attacker won't be.

You must get used to working from a position of disadvantage. Put yourself and your students in the worst positions you can (face down, under a bench, blindfolded to simulate blood in the eyes, and with an arm tied in their belt) and start the training from there. No "do-overs." Work from the position you find yourself in. There is no "right" move anyway, just moves that worked or didn't that one time.

When training for a position of disadvantage, be sure to stage the attacker close, as close as he would be in a real attack where the bad guy has chosen the optimum range.

Contact-response training. Condition for a quick, effective response to any unexpected aggressive touch. Trained properly, the counterattack will kick in *before* the chemical cocktail of stress hormones. This will give one technique at 100%, and possibly the initiative, to the expected victim. This level of conditioning is one of the few training methods that can address the suddenness of an assault. See next section on "Operant Conditioning" for the mechanism, but contact response training can harness the flinch into a counterattack, one of the few responses that can turn the tables. Flinches aren't telegraphed and they aren't bungled by thinking too much.

Train to flip the switch. Make your students practice going from friendly, distracted, or any other emotion to full-on in an instant. Make them play music, converse, fold clothes, write, or pour tea as an armored assailant attacks. The key is that the distraction must be natural and relaxed, not the jerky half-preparation of someone who expects an attack. The Reception Line Drill described later in Section 6.5 is an introduction to this concept. It may be an unrealistic expectation, but the goal of training in this aspect is to eventually make the alert, responsive, combative mind the norm. This also helps with the suddenness of the attack.

In slow-motion training, use realistic time framing. Do not let them pretend that "Monkey plucks jade lotus and presents to golden Buddha" is one move; do not let them pretend that a spinning kick is just as fast as a jab. Slow-motion training is a valuable tool, but not if students do things in training that they physically can't do at speed.

Get used to being hit, and get used to being touched, especially on the face. For various reasons, face contact between adults is loaded with connotations. Accidental face contact almost always results in both students freezing and can cause an outpouring of emotional sludge. Criminals use this by starting with an open-hand attack to the face (called a "bitch slap") that has paralyzing *psychological* effects.

Teach common sensitivity. They must respond to what is happening, not to their expectations or fears. If there are weapons mounted on the walls of your *dojo* and you are practicing self-defense, someone should be reaching for the weapons or running for the door. Some day, I will be teaching a roomful of Law Enforcement Officers (LEOs) and I will have an assistant rack a shotgun offstage. I will then ask the students who recognized the sound and all the hands will go up. I will then say, "So why are you still here? Are you stupid? Someone you don't know just loaded a shotgun right around the corner."

Forbid giving up. Winning is a habit. Fighting is a habit. Put them in positions where they are completely immobilized and helpless and set the expectation to keep fighting.

Adapting the four basic truths to your training. Sensei Kris Wilder, a Goju stylist in Seattle, has analyzed the four basic truths and turned them around. He says that everything he and his students do should serve to increase power and/or increase speed and/or close or at least better the position and/or contribute to surprise and the psychological advantage.

section 5.4: operant conditioning

Operant Conditioning (OC) is a system of training where a stimulus is matched to a response by reward. It is extremely powerful and can be done subtly or overtly; the results can be chosen or subconscious. Some would argue that all learned behaviors follow this model.

The elements of OC are the *stimulus*, which is whatever triggers the action; the *response*, which is what the subject does; and the *reward* or *punishment*, which is the direct result.

The stimulus can either be a single, simple thing or a collection of complicated things. For instance, a teacher may want to condition a rising block as a response to the stimulus of a straight punch to the face, or condition a multipurpose entry to any sudden movement from the front. Conditioning discrete responses to discrete stimuli is time-consuming, involved, and can never cover every eventuality—but it is simple. Conditioning a discrete response to a collection of related stimuli is slightly more difficult, but effective.

Martial arts training is heavy on response. By OC standards, everything you do, all actions, are responses. Even your best untele-graphed attack is a response to an opening.

Rewards are anything that increase the behavior. They can be as simple as a smile, a nod, or a grunt. A *positive* reward is something added to the system that tends to increase the behavior such as praise or food. A *negative* reward is the removal of something unpleas-ant. Heroin abuse is initially rewarded by the positive reward of the euphoric high. Later in the addiction cycle, it is negatively rewarded by the removal of withdrawal symptoms.

A punishment is anything that tends to decrease the behavior. A *positive* punishment is the addition of something, such as pain, to the system. A *negative* punishment is taking away something in order to decrease behavior. Spanking is positive punishment. Grounding is negative punishment.

Positive and negative in the context of OC are not value judgments and are not intended to modify the concept of reward and punishment. Rewards increase behavior regardless of what the reward is; punish-ments decrease the behavior—if it does not decrease the behavior, it is not a punishment by OC standards. Positive and negative refer only to whether something is given or taken.

In college, I trained a rat to push a lever. The system is to get a thirsty rat and put him in a cage with a lever and a waterspout. The lever is constructed so that if it is pushed, it makes a click and releases a drop of water at the spout. I also had a control switch that could make the click and release the water.

If the rat had just been left in the cage, he might have accidentally pushed the lever before he died of thirst, and he might not. He might have pushed the lever and never made the connection to the action and the appearance of water. My job was to train him to make the connection.

The key was that if he moved towards the lever, I pushed my but-ton. *Click.* Water. This is important. If you wait for your student to be perfect before rewarding, you will be waiting a long time. Reward any improvement.

If the rat only moved to the same place, I would reward a few more times and then stop. He had to move even closer to the lever than before to get water. This system of successive approximation (getting a little closer each time) quickly got the rat pushing the lever himself.

As an example, I emphasize contact/response training for ambush survival. For attacks from behind, I use the stimuli group "any unexpected, aggressive touch." So hair grabs, shoulder grabs, strikes to the head, neck, or kidneys, and attempts to take away holstered weapons are all treated the same.

The response is to drop-step and spin into the contact with an elbow lead. By repetition of the stimulus response pair and consistent reward as the students approach proficiency, the response can be brought up to nearly reflex speed.

section 5.5: the whole enchilada

Most martial arts are just a piece of the puzzle. Technically, some practice striking, some throwing, some practice both. Some add grappling and others specialize there. A truly complete martial art would cover everything from talking to shooting, and more besides.

Here is a training blueprint broken down by time, things you need to know if you ever defend yourself. Most will be touched on in this book, but seek further training in any aspect for which you are unprepared.

Training Phase 1: Long Before the Assault. Before anything bad happens, preferably years before, you should become familiar with the legal aspects of self-defense—how much force you can legally use, when you can use it, and when to stop.

You also need to work out your moral and ethical issues with regard to violence. This is discussed briefly in Section 6.2. If you can't shoot a human being, or couldn't blind one or are terrified of being crippled, you need to know this before you are in a position where it is possible or likely.

Training Phase 2: Before the Assault. Before anything bad happens, you need to understand how to avoid and prevent attacks.

Understand terrain. Develop awareness. Study predator, crime, and violence dynamics. Learn how to de-escalate someone verbally and learn the warning signs when it is too late to make de-escalation work. And don't get hung up here—a true predator won't give you a chance to use this level.

Training Phase 3: Operant Conditioning. Optimally, you need to train a small group of counterattacks to sudden assault and train them to reflex speed. This is one of the few things that can derail a predator's plan. If you have trained it well, this response will kick in before you freeze.

Training Phase 4: Breaking the Freeze. If you get hit and you weren't expecting it, you will almost certainly freeze. As described earlier, you need to recognize the freeze and act. If you do not, you will be stuck here. Game over.

Training Phase 5: The Fight. Everything you learned in martial arts now applies—if you got here. Phases 3 and 4, in my experience, are usually neglected in martial arts training. They are critical to keeping you functional long enough to access your training.

Remember, also, that you are fighting the threat's mind as well as his body.

Training Phase 6: The Aftermath. There may be legal consequences. There may be health issues and injuries. In a high end use of force, where someone is killed or crippled, there will almost certainly be emotional affects. Whether you did something or nothing. Whether you did right or wrong. Learn about these now.

Realistically, does your training address all six phases? If not, take the time to do the research or seek out the teachers who can help fill the holes. It's better not to fight at all. If you are a good fighter, you still need to survive to access your skills. Even then, if you aren't prepared for the consequences and turn to suicide or the slow-motion suicide of drugs or alcohol, you've still lost.

Learn the phases because no matter how skilled you are, failing at any one of the six can end you.

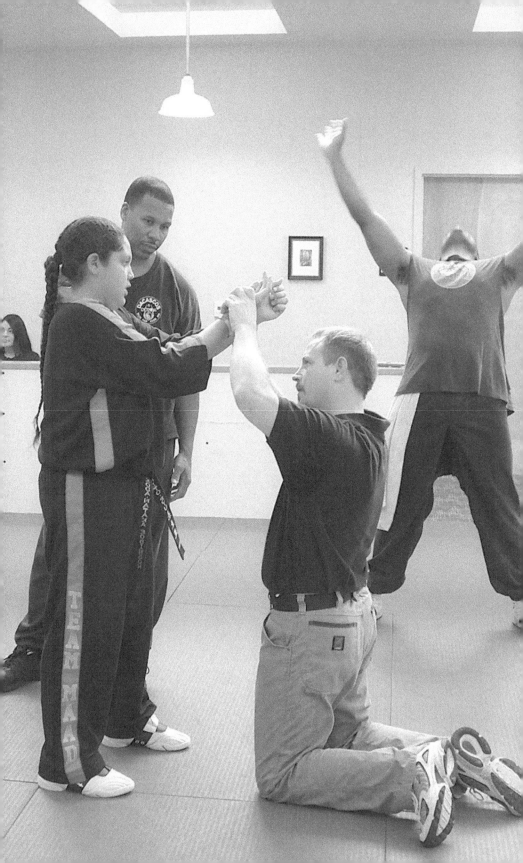

CHAPTER 6: MAKING PHYSICAL DEFENSE WORK

section 6.1: stages of defense: movement-opportunity-intent-relationship-terrain

Overview. There are five stages at which you can defend yourself from an assault. Most martial artists begin at Level 1, "blocking the motion." The fist comes in; the gun comes online. Because of the action/reaction gap, your chances of successfully blocking an already initiated attack are very low. Furthermore, blocking the attack does nothing to prevent a second or third attack. An encounter can only be won on the attack and defending puts you behind the curve.

Most martial artists then progress to Level 2, "blocking the opportunity." From an awareness of your available target areas and your threat's available weapons, you can reliably tell where an attack will come from, so you can prevent the move before it starts (this is how a good technician consistently beats your fastest attacks).

Many practitioners talk about Level 3, but few practice "blocking the intent." The pre-emptive strike. When you know or believe that the threat has decided to hurt you, you attack. It is the most effective physical defense but takes great skill to use and justify. Marc MacYoung, in *The Professional's Guide to Ending Violence Quickly,* did a very good job of writing down the signs that violence was imminent.

More effective still is Level 4, "altering the relationship." If you understand the dynamic (predator/prey, domestic violence cycles, dominance games, etc.), you can often prevent violence by altering the relationship between you and the threat. You can choose not to play the Monkey Dance. You can alter your appearance, habits, and

Correcting at seminar
Courtesy Kamila Z. Miller

mannerisms to not look like prey. You can get out of abusive relationships. Here, more than at any other stage, it is critical to understand that violence does not happen out of context. The goal at Level 4 is to change that context.

Lastly, Level 5, is the use of *terrain*. All violent encounters happen in places. There are places where violent encounters are common, others where they are very rare. Train yourself to be aware of ambush zones, escape and evasion routes, threat concentrations, etc. The ideal is to not be where the violence is likely to happen.

The bus let me off a half mile or so from my house about half-past midnight. It wasn't a particularly good part of town and we hadn't lived there very long, so in many ways it was unfamiliar terrain. I was young, happy. New job as a corrections deputy that I was enjoying, and going home to a wife I loved and a new baby.

Two men stepped out in front of me, blocking the sidewalk on a dark residential street. The smallest, who was still bigger than me, started a conversation and moved in close while his big brother hung back a little bit. I put on a smiley face and tried a friendly, "Don't have time now, guys. I'm on the way home." The smaller one put his hand on my chest and I gently parried it to the side.

"Don't fucking touch me," he snarled, and the big one swung. He hit the corner of my head, probably hurting his hand more than he hurt me. I backed up to the fence and put my hands up. Then a thought crossed my mind, a little whisper of a thought that changed many, many things. I remembered I was still on probation at the first real job in my life and for the sake of my wife and baby, I needed the job and the insurance. In a few heartbeats, I convinced myself that if I hurt either of these guys I would be fired.

In a two-on-one assault where I was attacked first, I made the potentially fatal and stupid decision not to hurt them.

Things happened fast. The big one struck again and I kicked him in the chest to knock him out of range. I thought, for some reason, that if they could see that I was fast, that I could kick faster than the big one could punch, they would back off. Instead, what they saw was that I didn't want to hurt them.

In the next flurry, I grabbed the big one and took him down. I'd intended a *sumi-gaeshi* and wound up in a tangle with him on top. He went to gouge my eyes and I wrapped the arm with my legs, both pushing him away from my eyes and putting his arm in a lock. I started to yell to his brother, "Back off or I'll break his arm!" That was my plan. Next time you are at the *dojo*, see how many times you can kick something on the floor in the time it takes to yell that simple phrase. I remember three of the kicks to the head pretty distinctly.

I rolled him off as quickly as I could and got to my feet. In the whole incident, the only serious damage I took was from those kicks and that was pretty cosmetic. The younger one backed off as I stood. I'm not sure why. He'd picked up my gym bag and swung it at my head. I stepped in and threw him with an *o-goshi*.

I remember standing there, bleeding, with my face swelling up thinking, "This is going pretty well."

It went on for about fifteen minutes before the police showed up. That was such a long time that twice the two brothers were winded and stopped attacking to chat with me...even suggesting that I go back to their house with them so that we could "finish this." That was the only possible stupid thing I didn't do that night.

By the numbers.

5—Terrain. If I hadn't been there, none of this would have happened. A different, more public route, better alertness, more aware of ambush zones and escape routes—any of these things could have saved a lot of damage.

4—Relationship. If I'd been able to alter the relationship, the attack could have been prevented with no damage. I did try, with the smiley-faced, "Don't have time now, guys. I'm on the way home." Many other tacks might have worked, or might have failed. It's a decade and a half later. I won't second-guess now.

3—Intent. It was obvious what was happening when they triangulated out to hem me in against the fence and the smaller one went to put his hand on my chest. They'd shown intent, but I wasn't prepared to take that as my "Go" button and explode into action. A pre-emptive attack at that time, which would have been justified, would have been my best physical chance at ending it with minimal damage to myself.

2—*Opportunity.* When I kicked the big one to show that I was faster, I used an awareness of opportunity. I knew another big overhand right was coming at my head and I knew he would be wide open. It worked for one attack, but did nothing to change the situation.

1—*Movement.* I remember the kicks coming at my head, but keying in on the motion there was nothing I could do about them in time. There rarely is in a real attack.

(1) **Responding to movement.** Many people are raised on fantasy ideas of speed and myths of "the fastest gun." In our Uncontrolled Environments Training, we have Simunitions weapons (real semiautomatic handguns that fire subcaliber marking rounds) and HighGear armor. During the class, I will hold a Sim gun at my side and let two deputies point their weapons at my chest, ready to fire. The deputies are instructed to order me to drop the weapon and to fire if I make any threatening move. They don't have to aim, they are locked on—fingers on trigger. I have to raise my weapon and fire. They only have to twitch a finger.

Consistently, I get off three shots before the fastest deputy can fire. If I sidestep, I will shoot both deputies before they fire and when they do fire, they miss with the first rounds. Action beats reaction.

If someone makes the decision to hit you and your first clue is the fist coming at you, you are responding to movement. The bad guy has sent a neural impulse from the brain to his muscles and the muscles are moving.

On the receiving end:
- The eyes (or ears or skin) sense the motion, they send an impulse down the nerves at about 200 fps (feet per second) to the brain.
- The brain interprets the perception.
- The brain chooses a response.
- The brain sends a signal at 200 fps down the nerves to the muscles...at this fourth step in the process, you are just getting to where the bad guy started.

There are ways to speed up each step, except nerve impulse travel. Peripheral vision, sound, and touch all have faster reaction times than focused sight.

Experience allows a more rapid interpretation of the perception. This can also be reversed with the technique of cognitive disruption, doing or saying something so unusual that it doesn't fit into any expected pattern.

On a late-night shift, one of our psych inmates told a nurse that all officers were vampires and that he was certain that we were going to come into his room in the middle of the night and kill him. Given that information, I would have slid a clove of garlic under his door and waited for daylight. The nurse, however, decided that officers had to enter the cell and bring the inmate to another area of the jail for closer observation.

That left us with medical instructions to act exactly like the inmate's delusions. Can you think of anything more likely to provoke a fight with a crazy guy?

I went into the cell with only a lieutenant for back-up. I stayed calm, kept a distance, and instructed the poor guy to get dressed. He was obviously terrified. He finally shrieked, "No! You're vampires!" and set himself to fight.

I said, "Nope. I'm part gypsy. Gypsies can't be turned to vampires."

He said, "What?" and froze. So did the lieutenant, by the way. They both clearly thought I was crazier than the crazy guy...didn't matter. I got cuffs on him before he could break out of the freeze.

The third step, when the brain chooses a response, is often the slowest step. The more options available, the bigger the "decision tree," the slower the decision tends to be. If you know eight good responses to a situation, choosing the best will take longer than if you only know one. For sudden attacks, I've trained my decision tree down to a "decision stick"—I have one response tied to any aggressive action I see. Nothing to think about. I have a different action if I feel it before I see it.

Simple pairings (if you see any movement from front, do X) are easier to train to near-reflex speed than complex pairings (if he swings with his right hand, do Y, if left hand, do Z; and if he kicks, do Q). *See* Section 5.4, Operant Conditioning.

(2) **Responding to opportunity is jumping ahead of the motion.** Move on the motion you know is coming rather than wait for it to happen. Stan Miller, the Pacific North West representative for Wally Jay's Small Circle Jujitsu, demonstrates a technique where he initiates a series of fast punches towards his opponent's face...and finger locks the opponent. "It's really reliable," he notes, "Even trained, closed-fist strikers, like boxers, open their hands and go palm-out when something unexpected goes at their eyes." Stan is a finger-lock specialist. When that hand opens, Stan is waiting for it. The fingers move into his grip, he's ahead of the curve.

It's easy to describe this in sparring terms. From any given position, there are only a few natural ways to move. If all your weight is on your right leg, you can only kick with your left. If you are leaning back at the same time, it has to be a front kick. Your knowledge of body mechanics, combined with your awareness of your own open targets, allows you to predict the most likely attacks and counter them.

Sparring, however, is not assault. Often, when this level of defense is used properly, the event is over. By properly, I mean aggressively counterattacking. Once an inmate, a short, stocky rapist, swung at my head. I'd known it was going to happen and I knew he would swing with his right hand. I jumped in and grabbed his hair, spinning hard to my right, and bringing him to the ground on his face.

(3) **Responding to intent.** Often, this boils down to a pre-emptive attack. Many, many people have problems with this concept. We've talked about action and reaction. For now, know this: *The first attack usually gets in.* The attacks that get in do damage. Each bit of damage you take hampers your ability to prevent more damage.

If you let the threat move first, you cede the initiative and, following the logic above, you take a step closer to your own failure.

You are an excellent judge of human behavior. You have been a human being for your entire life and have spent most of that life around other humans. Every human is an excellent judge of human behavior unless they willfully or unconsciously sabotage their own intuition. Want to know how good your human judgment is? How often have you been able to tell that someone was about to cut in front of you in traffic? You know this with no clues beyond a silhouette of the back of their head and the make and color of their car.

When you know that something is going to go bad, *move*.

Leaving is always good and defending at this level does not require an attack, it requires an action. If, as things are, you believe you are going to be attacked, you must change the way things are. Move, scream, run or fight, but do something. I've had excellent success with a sudden scream. I've tackled arrestees who reached for their pockets in certain ways. When three young men spread out to corner me, I started twitching rhythmically and holding a three-way conversation with Jesus and Elvis. They chose not to engage because crazy people are unpredictable.

(4) **Altering the relationship works on many levels.** Different types of violence exist in different social dynamics, but they all exist within a social framework.

Sometimes, as in stalking and predatory violence, the relationship is one-sided. The threat may have stalked, researched, and developed a detailed fantasy about the victim and the victim is completely unaware, but the relationship exists.

In abusive spouses and parenting, the relationship must change because the people won't. The abusive intimate relationship follows a particular pattern and it is foolish to think that a new stage in this cycle is a change in the person. End the relationship, or risk one of the people being ended. This is far too big a subject to cover here and my experience with it is limited.

Monkey Dance violence is predicated on the idea that there is a contest for dominance or social status between two people. If one of them refuses to play the game, pretending to be unaware of the challenge, the situation often evaporates.

"Whatchu lookin' at?"

"Was I staring? Damn, sorry about that. It's your shirt, dude. My ex-girlfriend got me one just like it. God, I hated that shirt."

Or (inmate in a separation cell): "Let me out of here, mother-fucker!" (kicking on the cell door), "Let me out right now or I'll fucking kill you!"

I opened the door, "What's your goal today, partner?"

"Huh?" (To be fair, when I opened the door he suspected he was going to get his ass kicked for making threats, so being nice gave me the advantage of surprise.)

"I said, what's your goal? What do you want to accomplish today?"

"I want to get out of this fucking cell and get out of jail."

I nodded. I was leaning up against the door in a stance I call the "modified Columbo"—left forearm in front of my ribs, right elbow resting on left wrist, right hand scratching my jaw thoughtfully. "That sounds reasonable. So tell me how screaming and threatening people is supposed to get you out."

"Huh?"

"You want to get out, right? And as far as the cell part goes, I'm the one you have to convince, so how does screaming and banging convince me to let you out?"

"Oh." Long pause. "You have a point."

"The RECOG* lady is a civilian. She's the one who will decide if you can get out tonight. If you scare her, do you think she's going to want you out on the streets or in jail?"

He nodded. "Probably in jail."

*Author's note: Some of these conversations are not going to be examples of scintillating wit. A lot of criminals aren't bright and many are locked into behavior patterns established as toddlers. If tantrums work, toddlers keep doing them. If tantrums turn into more violent expressions in a bigger child and they **still work** (e.g., the threat gets what he wants), violence will continue. Many of them are locked into a behavior pattern and have never, on their own, examined if it was working or not.*

---

*RECOG decides if an inmate can be "released to their own recognizance," essentially let out of jail with just a promise to make it to court.

"So you need to not scare her."

"That's right. You gonna let me out, Sarge?"

"Show me you can be quiet for an hour on your own. Deal?"

"Okay. Thanks, man."

Some predators use social skills to get close to their victims. I recommend Gavin DeBeckers book, *The Gift of Fear* for excellent and detailed descriptions of the techniques used. Read the book, but I'll summarize two concepts:

Charm is a verb. People are not charming; charm is something they use to get what they want. When someone attempts to use charm, ask yourself what they want. It might be bad.

Don't be afraid to be rude. In the vast majority of these predatory assaults, you did not ask for the attention and you have no obligation to the person trying to get close, no matter what he tells you or what your momma told you about being polite.

The predator who works off the blitz, the sudden overwhelming attack, chooses his victims carefully. The best defense, at this stage, is to look and act like someone who would be a very expensive victim, someone who would make an attacker pay. It is projecting confidence and self-value.

I could go and repeat everything you've ever heard about posture, body language, and eye contact but they would just be words. Soon, while these words are fresh in your mind, go to a bar, take a ride on a bus, or walk in a crowded park, fair, or market. First, look at the crowd like a predator would. If you needed to get money, soon and at the least risk to yourself, who would you attack? How? Where? There are people in every crowd looking at you exactly that way. Start training yourself to see what they see. Look at it from the blitz point of view: Who appears weak, unaware, or sick? Who is self-effacing with bad posture? Who is alone? Who is too drunk to respond to an attack?

Who could you get close to? Is there a child who looks too eager to please or desperate for attention? A frazzled, distracted mother? An older lady carrying groceries who would be grateful for the assistance of a "gentleman"?

Look at these victims—and don't act like them. Just as it is hard to look at your own assumptions, it is also hard to evaluate your demeanor. Look at yourself, have friends and instructors you trust evaluate you, and look in a mirror or use a video.

Conversely, look at the exact same crowds and identify the people you WOULDN'T mess with. Let your gut identify them first. If your intellect gets into it, you will look for big, strong people. Your gut will identify the ones with confidence and dedication, and a will to live. It will identify the crazy, the committed, and the experienced.

Imitate these people. Look at how they stand and dress and position themselves in a room. How they hold eye contact and with whom and for how long. How they walk and use their hands and talk and listen.

(5) **Use of terrain is the highest order of defense because if you aren't there, you can't even get your feelings hurt.** It's nothing quite so banal as "Don't walk down dark alleys alone," but damn, that's good advice.

Bad things happen in places. Bad things are done by bad people. If you avoid the bad people and bad places, you usually avoid the bad events.

Avoiding dangerous places is the *strategic* level of terrain. *Tactically*, you have to learn to read and use the terrain around you. Notice places where you can be cut off, trapped, or surrounded. Identify exits and objects that can be used for cover and concealment. Who can see you? Who can see better than you can? If a window looks like a mirror to you, people on the other side can see in just fine.

Develop the habit of planning for escape and evasion (E&E), because not being there is always the best solution. In the room you are in right now, and every room you enter until it becomes second nature, notice every way out—every door, every window you can break; every grill in the floor, wall, or ceiling.

Notice your routes to those exits, what cover and concealment is available to those routes, and from which direction you are covered. Concealment, for our purposes, is anything that can keep the threat from seeing you. Cover is anything that can stop a bullet. Distance can work for both.

Eventually, work into the habit of not only knowing all the exits from the room you are in, but where the exits lead. There is no excuse for not knowing in intricate detail how to navigate the buildings you spend much time in—your home, office, and favorite recreational areas. Read the little fire escape maps when you check into a hotel or go to a new building for a meeting.

Also use terrain and the environment offensively. Catalog all the items in your pockets and within your reach that can be used for weapons. How would you use them? Pay attention to low furniture, bad footing, table edges, and doorknobs that can work as striking or tripping services.

I was eighteen and trying to talk a friend into joining the Judo team at OSU. Robby was short, strong, and had an incredibly devious mind. I thought he'd be perfect for competition Judo. We sat in his living room, drinking across a messy coffee table. He was on the couch, I was opposite him in a chair.

"Nah," He said.

"You'd love it—it's fun, good exercise, and good self-defense."

"Nah. I'd never need any of that martial arts bullhockey."

"What do you mean?"

Robby gave his snotty little grin. "That's for stupid people. I don't need it."

He'd pissed me off just a little. "What's that supposed to mean?"

"Rory, only stupid people get into fights. Only the really stupid ones think that fighting skill will get 'em out. The smart guy always wins."

"Bull. What if I attacked you right now?" (You all see where this is going, right?)

"Go ahead."

I stood up and the little weasel kicked the corner of the coffee table into my shin. When I started the one-legged hopping, he used a pillow from the couch and smacked me with it, catching me perfectly off-balance. I went down.

Robby snickered, "Told you. Fighting is for stupid people."

Author's note: The smart guy doesn't always win, doesn't even usually win—but an exceptionally sneaky, cunning, cold-blooded person can get away with some things. I've learned a lot from Robby over the years.

Repeating myself: It's better to avoid than to run; better to run than to de-escalate; better to de-escalate than to fight; better to fight than to die. The very essence of self-defense is a thin list of things that might get you out alive when you are already screwed.

This rest of this chapter will be about fighting and not dying.

section 6.2: the "go" button

If you are ever faced with extreme violence, you will have to make the decision to act. Make it now. You must decide what is worth fighting for, never forgetting that the question involves the risk of both dying and killing. You must decide now. Taking damage in the middle of a shitstorm of fists and boots is the wrong time to agonize over the moral dimension of conflict. There are things worth fighting for. List what they are.

Once you have made the list, these are your "Go" buttons. You must commit that if one of them happens you will act ruthlessly and decisively. You cannot second-guess yourself in the moment.

Here are some examples:
- I will always act if someone attempts to tie or handcuff me.
- If someone threatens a child with a weapon.
- If someone attempts rape.
- If someone tries to move me to a secondary crime scene.
- If a lone armed threat puts down his weapon and either the threat or the weapon is within arm's reach.
- If I see an exit and the threat is not focused on me.

Some of these are intellectual. I've evaluated my odds and consciously chosen them. If a criminal attempts to move me someplace where he is less likely to be disturbed (a secondary crime scene), there are no good possible results. There are no positive benefits to a violent criminal wanting to have a long stretch of time alone with me.

Some are emotional. I've counseled a number of rape victims. I would rather do something with a very low chance of success or survival than wake up every morning with the memory that I did nothing.

If the "Go" button hits, I will fight or run...I will do something. The plan may be made in the instant or in the moments leading up to the precipitator, but the "Go" button is the trigger.

For the record, someone trying to kill you had damn well better be one of your "go" buttons.

section 6.3: the golden rule of combat

This section is about fighting, ways to efficiently work that choice. This book is not a manual. I have techniques, tactics, and strategies that have worked for me and that I trust; this section will be about understanding the techniques you have been taught and what makes them efficient or inefficient.

In an old book on *Kano* Jujitsu, I found the "The Golden Rule of Combat." I've never seen it elsewhere and I can't find the book again, so I can't even properly credit it, but it is the best advice on finishing a combat that I've ever seen.

The Golden Rule of Combat:
Your most powerful weapon
Applied to your opponent's greatest vulnerability
At his time of maximum imbalance

Your best shot at his weakest point when he's least ready. The three elements: Power Generation, Targeting, and Timing.

Power Generation. Theodore Roosevelt said, "The unforgivable crime is soft hitting. Do not hit at all if it can be avoided; but never hit softly." I occasionally have to take a bad guy down and put cuffs on without hurting him. In a self-defense situation, the whole concept of not hurting should be alien.

Most martial artists work very hard on power generation. They have mastered rotational power; conducting energy from the legs to the fist through a solid base; using relaxation and tension at appropriate times. All good. Some have worked on using gravity and body weight as a speed and power multiplier. This skill is essential for small people. If your current training doesn't incorporate it, seek someone who can teach it.

Possibly the most overlooked aspect of power generation in the martial arts is one of the most effective: Use a tool. I will take a hickory baseball bat over the hardest fist on Okinawa. A weapon extends reach, increasing power, leverage, and speed. You don't break your metacarpals when you hit with a phone or a padlock in a sock. Tools are everywhere, limited only by your imagination and experience.

The most effective unarmed practitioner will consistently lose to a mediocre practitioner who has a weapon.

Continuous striking is another power multiplier. Be very careful in training not to develop the habit of striking once or twice and then pausing to gauge the effect. Even police officers are trained to shoot until the threat goes down. When you are already the victim and close enough to be in arm's reach, it is even more critical. If you must attack, keep the attack on until the threat is no longer capable of harming you.

Attack hard. Attack ferociously. "Violence of Action Trumps Technique"—Deputy U.S. Marshal Jeff Jones. Hitting hard, fast, and aggressively is more effective that hitting properly. Both are good, but violence of action wins.

Be cautious with gloved sparring. Gloves encourage closed-fist strikes to the head and real hands tend to break when they do that. They also rely on multiple micro-concussions to get an effect, sometimes leading to a pushing style of striking, which delivers less damage with bare hands than a snap. Gloves are good tools for learning to strike a moving body hard. My personal solution has been to use armor and no gloves. You still get used to hitting a moving target hard, but you can't get as lazy with your hand conformation.

Targeting. You hit the places where it will have the most effect as hard as you can. My preference is to shut down the brainstem, attack the knee of the leg with the most weight on it, over-pressure the ears, collapse the throat, and shock or rupture the liver with strikes. I attack the spine, collarbone, knees, and elbows for unbalancing and immobilizations. This will be very dependent on your training.

Be careful of training where the targets are ineffective or non-specific. A strike to the chest is worthless against a much larger opponent, where a strike to the solar plexus on the chest might be effective.

Timing. Though timing is one of the most critical and complex of sparring skills, it is a very simple thing in self-defense. There are two good times to hit someone:

When you have no choice, *and,*

When you can get away with it.

You have no choice when you are taking damage or about to take damage or be restrained. When the options to run or hide don't exist and there is no discretionary time, you attack. It's a bad situation and even under the full adrenaline dump that leaves you flailing blindly, it is better than standing there.

If you have discretionary time, you attack when you can get away with it. If the threat looks away or puts down his weapon or reaches for a drink, you attack. In a long-term hostage situation where you have successfully personalized and the threat starts to trust you, you strike. You must strike hard, fast, and with total commitment.

section 6.4: effects and actions

There are four combative physical effects you can have on your opponent:

1. You can move him, or part of him
2. You can cause pain
3. You can cause damage, or
4. You can cause shock

Movement is simple. At its crudest level, it is using muscle power to push or pull someone around. It is used to create space, deny space, create distance, immobilize, increase damage, or decrease damage.

Create space. In a tight, close-range fight especially on the ground, there is an art to creating space for you to move. It can involve clearing your own or the threat's limbs or body so that you have access to targets, or creating enough of a window that you can use a strike. It can involve creating space between you and the wall, ground, or another surface so that you can move, or suddenly opening a space that your opponent will fall into.

Deny space. Use your body and available objects to deny the threat free movement. A person standing has a complete sphere in which they can move. I take threats to the ground so that half of that mobility is cut off by the earth. The clinch in boxing is denying the opponent the free space to strike.

Create distance. Very often, getting away is the ultimate goal in an attack. If you can push or pull the threat in such a way that you have the space to sprint, you can do it. In this context, *space* is freedom of movement; *distance* is a chance to escape.

Immobilize. A pin is an immobilization, but there are other ways to use strength, balance, and leverage to stop a threat from moving or stop part of a threat, such as his fist or boot, from moving.

Increase damage. Strikes are more effective if the target is frozen in place. Strikes are even more effective if the target is being pulled in to them in a two-way action.

Decrease damage. Power can be bled off of strikes by maintaining contact with the striking limb or jamming the root of the limb. Try slamming a palm into an opponent's hip while he tries to knee kick. Damage can also be decreased by moving with the force, and most attacks will evaporate if the threat's balance can be suddenly disrupted.

I use wrestling as a model for this skill, but any grappling style will teach you how to move a body. Knowing how to move a body is critical, especially for people unfamiliar with the "closer" aspect of the Four Basic Truths (Section 3.2). Size helps, but the skills of applied power, balance, and timing can be learned and should be studied.

In real encounters, movement skills have the advantage of being independent of the threat's mental state. It does not matter if the threat is psychotic or drugged to the eyeballs, a sweep is still a sweep; if his center of gravity gets pushed outside of his base, he will stumble or fall. The disadvantage is that by itself, except for creating room to run, it can't end the encounter.

Pain. Pain is the physiological and psychological reaction to a *bad thing*. There are three legitimate uses for pain: as a negotiating tool, to trigger a predictable flinch response, or to stop the threat from thinking.

Pain is used as a negotiating tool very often in martial arts and in law enforcement. When an officer kneels on the jaw hinge or grinds a knuckle into the mastoid nerve and yells, "Quit resisting!" it is actually a simple deal: if the threat cooperates with the process, the pain will stop. In martial sports, the joint lock submission is a negotiation for surrender. In order for pain to work as a negotiating tool, the threat must be able to understand your verbal commands.

Certain pains have very specific flinch or movement response associated with them. These can be used to create space in a certain place or to set up secondary moves. I use one in the forearm combined with one in the jaw to set up my favorite sweep.

A sudden, sharp pain can completely blot out the conscious mind. It can cause a moment of hesitation or freezing that can be exploited. In certain cases, it can tip the person over the edge into fight/flight survival mode, which can be good if they run or bad if they frenzy.

Punishment. There is, in addition to the three legitimate uses above, a fourth use. Punishment, in this context, is an attempt to make someone a better person by hurting them. It is a perversion of the punishment of operant conditioning and sometimes people fall into the temptation. You cannot make a criminal better through pain. You can make them fear you. You only confirm their worldview: those who can hurt, hurt; the strong get what they can take; you hurt those weaker than you. A blind attempt at punishment, "I'm gonna teach you a lesson, boy," only teaches a criminal to be more careful and more brutal with a series of weaker victims.

In self-defense, pain is always an extra, NEVER the primary goal of a technique. Some people can focus through pain. Many threats under the influence of drugs, alcohol, or mental illness are completely immune to pain.

Damage. Damage is destroying structural integrity to the point that all or part of the body is not useable. In your training, be very careful that you understand the difference between pain and damage. As a guest at a Kung Fu school, I was sparring with one of their senior belts. It was friendly, non-contact stuff. At one point, my opponent suddenly stopped and said, "The custom in our school is for you to respond to a good hit like it was real."

"I thought I was."

"I just hit you in the nose," she said. "That would have broken it."

I was honestly puzzled. "Right, so I hit you back. That's what I did to the last two people who broke my nose." She had been taught that a good shot to the nose would end the fight.

A broken nose, while fairly painful, is not debilitating in any way. You can keep fighting through it and so could your opponent. Be aware that some can ignore damage to a limited degree—occasionally, you will run across someone who will punch with a broken hand — but not a shattered elbow. I did a Judo *randori* match after my ACL (anterior cruciate ligament) snapped. The knee had bent completely backward. I didn't do well, but I wasn't finished, either. Nothing is 100% reliable.

Shock. Shock is shutting down systems, usually by impairing the circulatory or nervous system so severely that the organism ceases to function. This does not necessarily mean death or even unconsciousness. A bullet to the head does result in shock, but so does a strangle, knocking the wind out, or lying on the lower ribs and letting the threat get tired. You can also shock parts of the body by cutting off blood or nerve impulses to limbs—not often practical, but nice to know. Cutting off blood supply works on everyone—regardless of drugs, rage, or size—which makes the strangles (*shime-waza*) the big equalizer.

The Effects and Actions concept is a powerful training tool. It is an intellectual way to introduce the practitioner into concepts of strategy and tactics. Martial artists and combatants can and should use certain

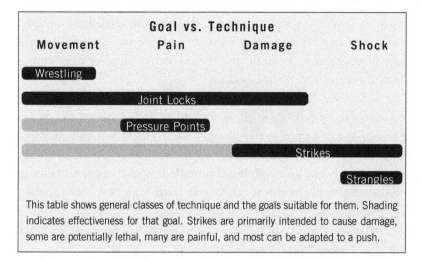

This table shows general classes of technique and the goals suitable for them. Shading indicates effectiveness for that goal. Strikes are primarily intended to cause damage, some are potentially lethal, many are painful, and most can be adapted to a push.

actions to get certain effects. This must be practiced for a long enough period of time in the training hall so that this intellectual and physical exercise becomes the "only natural way to move" when you need it.

section 6.5: the big three

In the end and at the deepest level, successful physical defense will depend on three things: Awareness, Initiative, and Permission. Each of these is a study in itself and can be a paradigm for combatives training. Together, they are the keys to exceptional performance in survival and in life.

Deputy Paul McRedmond introduced the concept of awareness-based training to me and to our agency. At the lowest level, it is simply that once you know what is going on with your body, the threat's body, the situation, and the environment—what you need to do becomes obvious. In this paradigm, techniques are not memorized but understood, and technique training becomes looking for opportunities

The system can be broken down in many ways and to many levels.

Awareness of your own body. Understanding your anatomical weapons and weaknesses—anatomy, physiology, and kinesthetics—

your own structure and movement patterns and tendencies. Simply, you have had your body your whole life. Unless you have been deliberately not paying attention, you are intimately familiar with what a human body is and does, especially yours.

Awareness of the opponent's body. All the same things apply because it is, despite drugs or rage, a human body with which you are dealing. You train through sight and touch to know not only what the body is doing now but what the body is about to do. As an easy drill, practice slow-motion infighting blindfolded. With a little practice you can sense actions the threat is about to make with only slight contact by reading shifts in balance and rotation around the spine.

Awareness of the situation. Enables you to accurately perceive and use the nuances of environment to your advantage.

Awareness of the dynamic. Recognizing the pre-assault cues so that you can prevent the situation. Dealing with the situation as it is, (e.g., recognizing the Monkey Dance for what it is or not deluding yourself that you can plead a process predator into changing his mind). This involves a ruthless dedication to dealing with the situation as it is, and not responding to either imagined fears or wishful thinking.

Awareness of your duty, your beliefs, and your place in the universe. Your "Go" buttons. An internal and deep understanding of what is worth fighting, dying, or killing for, what you can or can't do. Mauricio Machuca, an instructor in Montreal, talks about capability versus capacity. It is easy to teach someone how to break a neck. With a few minutes' training, a healthy person will have the technical and physical capability to break a neck, but very, very few could actually do it. They lack the capacity. Be aware of your capacity.

At a level I am just starting to understand now, much of what goes on in conflict is subject to a plethora of subconscious rules and unspoken contracts. I have found these affecting the amount of power that can be delivered, damage withstood, and time. Awareness of these rules and which are artificial is a huge advantage.

Initiative-based training was introduced to me by Deputy U.S. Marshal Jeff Jones. In any given situation, you can tell what needs to be done. Do it. Without hesitation, without wind-up, without telegraph, you act when it is time to act. It doesn't matter if it is not what you planned or things aren't going well. In each instant, something needs to be done and you do it.

Obviously, this predicates on being aware of what needs to be done, but it is a powerful training tool by itself. Hold a practice knife to a student's throat and tell them to do something about it, and then watch as they size up the situation, thinking about and discarding options, set their shoulders to move, then change their minds. When they finally move, you will see it coming with plenty of time to spare.

If and when they learn to act decisively, you won't see it coming; the movement will be explosive, hard, and un-telegraphed, and you will not have time to respond. Which movement they use is irrelevant. A slap, an entry, a kick, a lock, or a strike will all work. The technique is irrelevant. To quote Jeff, "Violence of action trumps technique."

At the technique level, this is acting decisively and without hesitation or telegraph, regardless of the technique used. At the tactical level, it is explosive entry. At the strategic level, it is "Shock and Awe." At the meta-level, it is deciding what is worth fighting, dying, or killing for long before the subject comes up, and acting decisively when the line is crossed—the second half of the "Go" button.

Like awareness, this can go deep and can affect far more of your life than simply combat or self-defense. Want to change your life forever? Commit right now to never make a half-assed decision again. Stay in bed or get up, but never again lay in bed thinking that you should get up. Jump in the water or don't, but never wade in slowly to get used to it.

In combat, if you are aware, you know what needs to be done. Do it. In life, you know what needs to be done, you know the right things to do. Do them.

Permission is my contribution to the Big Three, sort of. Years ago in Montreal at a symposium, I was presenting training to a small group of martial artists. I used the Reception Line Drill. In this drill, one student has been designated an important official who must attend a reception in his or her honor. That student stands in place and greets all of the other students as they pass by in a reception line. One of the other students, the "assassin," has a training knife and complete freedom on when and how to use it. The assassin can wait for the handshake and stab with the student's hand controlled, try for friendly hug, or wait until the line is nearly over and attack from behind. The original purpose of the drill was to train students to switch from friendly or social to fighting in an instant.

In Montreal that day, I saw some outstanding martial arts, but almost no real self-defense. No one yelled for help or warned others of the knife. No one ran for the door. No one took one of the many weapons lying around (it was, after all, a martial arts studio) and used it to defend themselves. This was a clue.

For a long time, I assumed that the issue was a lack of awareness, that the students got so caught up in the drill that they ignored everything that wasn't right in front of them. It never occurred to me that on some level they thought it wasn't allowed.

Irena originally tried Jujutsu because her Karate training hadn't included breakfalls. She stuck with it beyond the breakfall skill because of the different way Jujutsu looked at violence. She was a good *karateka* with good skill and excellent form. She could hit like a mule on the heavy bag...but she couldn't hit a person with the same power. She wouldn't let herself.

Sonia caught me good, a solid elbow in the mouth. She jumped away. "I'm sorry! Are you okay?"

"Yeah! That was great!"

"It was too hard."

"No it wasn't. It was exactly what you're supposed to do. I'm teaching you to hit people. I expect to get hit occasionally."

"I don't want to hurt you."

"Then you are really in the wrong class. Sonia, you have permission to hurt me. You're here to learn how to hurt someone." Another clue.

Dana Sheets provided the last clue to bring it all together by bringing an article to my attention, "Betrayed by the Angel: What happens when violence knocks and politeness answers?" by Debra Anne Davis published in the *Harvard Review* #26. In the article, Ms.

Davis describes her rape with great insight, poignancy, and brutal honesty. Throughout the article, she describes moments where she didn't want to be rude, where she didn't give herself permission to really resist.

Permission. With all the skill in the world, you must still let yourself act. If you need to hurt someone to survive, the first battle may be in your head. It has to be okay for you to hurt someone. A small woman with a little training can strike hard enough to break a rib or a clavicle, if she lets herself.

There is more. It's amazing how much of fighting is mental, how much is pure imagination, and how much is an unspoken agreement. Hollywood knockouts, where you get hit in the head and go to sleep for awhile and wake up fine don't occur in nature. If an animal gets hit hard enough in the head for it to go down, there's some serious damage. Same with focused people and people on drugs. I've taken a well-aimed hit with no loss of consciousness and been dizzy and puking for days.

But sometimes you give a light tap to a healthy person who has no stomach for the fight and he'll drop, convinced he's been "knocked out."

Like awareness and initiative, permission also works on many levels. Once you develop the awareness that certain rules are artificial, you can choose to break them. We noticed this first in grappling and locking—people have an instinct to fight against the place where they feel contact. While kneeling on a threat's arm, if the threat chooses to fight, he will do so by trying to use arm strength to lift the weight of the knee off. The lower leg, foot, and ground make a big triangle with a lot of space at the foot end when you are kneeling. The threat could escape at any time, easily, simply by yanking his hand toward the foot end of the triangle.

There are locks where the limb is controlled in exactly two places and can escape by any movement other then pressing against the two points of contact, but untrained people fight the force, not the emptiness. Trained people often don't generalize from skills they have (such as slipping wrist locks) to identical skills (such as slipping spine locks).

Further, some martial artists are trained to see things in a certain way, putting more imaginary rules on their actions than an untrained person. There is a hold that is sometimes taught as very difficult to escape from, that is easy as anything simply because I was caught in the hold and escaped from it before anyone could tell me it couldn't be done.

Playing with the concept in space, we found it applied to time, also. Any good fighter can tell you that he can control the tempo of an altercation. It's dangerous to do in real life, but I have slowed down and found the threat subconsciously slowing down to match me... and once with a PCP freak, I found myself accelerating beyond what I thought was my maximum speed to catch up.

Timing is one of the classic elements of dueling and sparring. It's simpler in a real fight but still critical. In my style, we emphasize getting and maintaining the initiative, taking the fight to the threat.

The Japanese phrase for this constant assault tactic is "Leaving no space for death to enter." Loren Christensen has phrased it as elegantly as possible: "There are so many beats in a fight. I want each of those beats filled up with *my* stuff." An overwhelming attack is a very, very reliable way to take out a threat. You take up all the time, leaving none for him.

This, too, is an agreement. Everyone in a battle has their own time and their time is all theirs. It can only be taken away if it is given up. You do not have to wait politely like a child trying to get a word in on a family argument. Try this with your students (safely): throw a flurry of chain punches or "rolling thunder" at their faces and watch them cover and, subconsciously, wait for their turn to respond. If the same rain of blows is coming at your face, there is nothing but your own mind keeping you from hitting back at the same time...but it does, and reliably enough that both predatory criminals and tactical entry teams count on it.

The Big Three are potent in combination.

Initiative and awareness in combination allow the predator dynamic. They allow the explosive counterattack that can save a victim from a hopeless situation. Together, they allow for devastating and explosive applications of skill that push the very edge of what is possible.

Permission and awareness go beyond that. There are agreements and subconscious human dynamics that affect violent behavior. Cultivating awareness of which of these agreements are artificial, and granting yourself permission to break them combine for a nearly superhuman ability. It is not that you can suddenly do what humans can't do, it's that you can do what humans choose to believe they can't do. Serious, skilled combative martial artists have said that small joint locks can't be used in a real fight, but I've done it, even one-handed on threats who outweighed me by a bunch. You will be told that if you go up unarmed against a threat with a knife, you will be cut, yet I stand at five enounters without a scratch. More importantly is context—the rule is that you cannot take someone down who is in excited delirium without a mass of officers or good weapons... but not only have I done it a couple of times I've talked even more down—I was aware that the context (excited delirium produces a frenzied rage and inability to listen or reason), close quarters, *et cetera*, dictated a certain kind of response ONLY if I agreed. I gave myself permission NOT to agree and turned fights into talks. NOT every time. Nothing is 100%.

Permission and initiative combine to produce a force of nature. This is inhuman and hard to describe. You do what needs to be done without regard for whether it is possible, because nine-tenths of your "impossibilities" are imaginary. Strange that a 110-pound girl believes that she can't hurt a 200 pound man, but an eight-pound cat (especially if you dump a bucket of water on it) can and will do so without hesitation. A small woman can punch hard enough to break ribs, and it is far less a matter of "know-how" than it is of deciding to injure and then letting herself do it. This, really, is what has allowed me to go up against PCP freaks—in the end, the critical difference between me and them is that they have completely lost their allegiance to regular human suppositions about what is and isn't true, is and isn't possible. They lose their sense of reality through chemicals, and sometimes I can give mine up and even the playing field.

Permission

This is something I give my students . . .

Sometimes I ask, "Why didn't you...?" reach for a weapon, use a preemptive strike, run, call for help...

And the student says, "I didn't know I could."

For the longest time, I assumed that meant the student had never considered it or didn't know how...it didn't occur to me that they thought it might be forbidden.

These are things that should never need to be said but still must, because there is power in the words.

- You have permission to defend yourself.

- You have permission to be rude.

- You have permission to survive, no matter what it takes.

- You have permission to act when the scary man reaches for his belt. You do not need to wait until he draws the weapon or until he points it at you, or until he hurts you. You have permission to act.

- You have permission to beat me, even if I wear a black belt.

- You have permission to become better than the best instructor you ever had.

- You have permission to invent something better than I ever taught you, permission to use it in my class, permission to use it to defeat me, and permission to teach it to your students.

- You have blanket permission to grow and live and survive and fight and run and scream and talk and play and laugh and learn and experiment. You have permission to win, and you have permission to decide what winning is. Be amazing!

—Rory

I very rarely talk about the "twilight zone" of violence, the incredibly weird things that happen, some seemingly impossible. One of those stories is about the time I saw a threat start to punch at my partner. Everything went in slow motion. I took two long steps, shoved my partner out of the way, and caught the fist in midair. By conventional wisdom, this was impossible. Action beats reaction, and I didn't start to move until after the threat had started the punch. In addition, you can't take two long steps and push someone out of the way in the time it takes him to throw a short left hook. But that one time I did. That experience has always been in the twilight zone—how the hell did that happen? How strange is that? Looking at it from this perspective, it was just permission and initiative, and the question becomes, "Why don't I do that all the time?"

Can this be taught and transmitted? I can give you permission to act and show you how a lock or a pin is an agreement and that works pretty well, but how well does it work when I tell you that you don't need to be a victim? That you can change your world? That you can do the impossible every day?

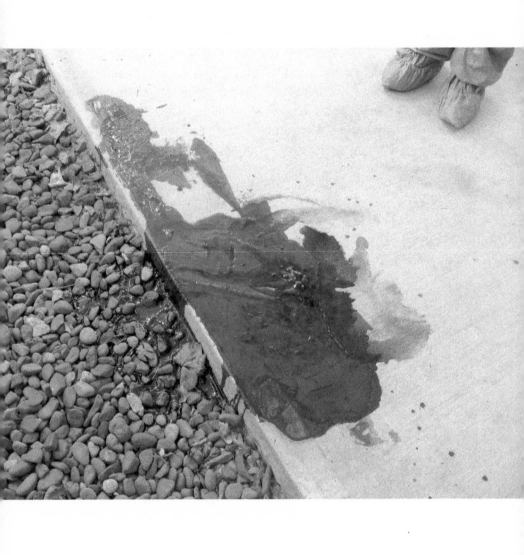

CHAPTER 7: AFTER

section 7.1: after

A lot of this book has been about the psychology of violence, the attacker, the defender, and the context of the attack; the psychology before and during the attack. Another psychology of violence deals with the aftereffects of violence.

Freud taught that sex and aggression were the two most powerful drives in the human psyche. He was wrong, of course. If you go for two days without sex and water, you will go for the water first when you get the chance. At the same time, he was very right. It's not that sex and violence are the two most powerful human drives, it's that sex and violence are the two areas where what we have been told is "right" and what we feel can have the greatest conflict. How we resolve these conflicts greatly defines our personality.

For many people, violence and their response to it is a staple of their fantasy life: from daydreams to movies, video games, and role-playing, and even to the extent of studying martial arts. They have an image of who they are and what they will do if ever faced with violence. This image is cultivated for years and is a very real aspect of self-identity. Very rarely does that fantasy survive contact with actual violence. It can be devastating.

Violence is not the same as danger. The fear of injury from rock climbing, parachuting, or kayaking is not the same as the fear of conflict. For most people, it is easier to engage in an endeavor where there is physical danger (real or perceived) than where there is social danger (real or perceived).

Take a person bungee jumping for the first time. Time how long it takes and how much encouragement it takes to get your friend to jump. A very few jump without hesitation. Most take some time to work themselves up to jumping. Very, very few can't jump at all.

Sidewalk blood
Courtesy Critical Care BioRecovery, LLC

Take the same person to a karaoke bar and see how long it takes him to work up the courage to sing. Other than people who have dedicated themselves to singing, it usually takes not only a good deal of time and encouragement, but also alcohol, bets, and name-calling to get someone on stage...but what is really at risk? How a bunch of drunken strangers will perceive them. Nothing more.

It is easier for most people to rappel for the first time than it is to ask an attractive stranger for a date (sober, anyway).

The danger from rappelling, rafting, climbing, skiing (real or perceived) is danger to the body, physical danger. It threatens your *life*. It is affirming for your identity.

There is no physical danger from singing or public speaking, but the fear is very real. These actions threaten your identity. They threaten your *self*.

In acts of violence, what the world *is* comes into direct conflict with what we expect the world *should be*. In acts of violence, your body and your self-image can both be damaged. It can be shattering. For most people, the event that shatters their identity beyond repair is also the event that takes their life. The tragic accident that killed the person also killed their feeling of invulnerability. The incurable disease kills the body and the naïve belief that "it will never happen to me." Surviving violence often leaves physical wounds that heal, but damages the person's basic beliefs and assumptions—about life, about other people and about themselves—to the extent that who they *were* no longer applies. They are alive. Their identity, this story that they have spent their entire life building, is shattered. It is not real, but that doesn't matter.

Some of fighting for social status is biology. Humans aren't well adapted to surviving alone. Half a million years ago, conflict in the group could endanger the whole group and was discouraged. Power plays and establishing one's rank in the hierarchy were critical but preferably subtle. An open conflict or direct challenge put the challenger at some risk of injury but even more at risk of being cast out, and that was certain death. You have a lot of hard-wiring to keep you from taking that risk.

I also believe that violence can be more psychologically damaging, partially because it has become so rare. For the majority of people in industrialized western civilization, violence will never touch their lives directly. This absence of a touchstone to reality allows the fantasies and daydreams to run and grow and spread.

The media has done a good job of convincing us that these are violent, dangerous times. They have convinced many that the past was a simpler and more peaceful era where wars were relatively civilized and serial killers were unknown. This is simply not true.

section 7.2: acute events

What will it be like if you survive a serious encounter? It will be like losing a tooth and you can't help poking at the hole. Whether it went well or not, you'll be playing it back again in your mind, over and over. Months later you may come up with something that might have worked better or prevented the whole thing, and you will feel guilty because it didn't occur to you in the quarter of a second it might have helped.

Many martial artists change schools or styles, looking for the silver bullet that will work next time. If it is never tested, they have the luxury of becoming fanatical about the new school. Some gave up training altogether because it didn't work. A very few make the decision that they will be ready next time and start to adjust their training to fit their experience. This is more rare than it should be. I have seen gifted martial artists teach that attacks happen in a certain specific and unrealistic way when they have actually survived assaults that were nothing like their models. I do not understand denial at this level, but it happens and is passed from instructor to student.

Another thing you need to know is that in a really bad situation (say someone dies or was raped), you will go through this no matter what you did. If you handled it perfectly and someone dies, justified all the way, you will go through this. If you made the situation worse, you will go through this. And if you did nothing, *especially* if you did nothing, you will go through this.

It's no big deal.

That probably sounds cold. *Humans are not machines that get broken and then get fixed.* Humans are creatures and something happens to them and they grow. They can grow twisted, true. But most grow stronger if they are allowed to.

I part company with many researchers on Post-Traumatic Stress Disorder here. This is from the heart, from my own experience. Take it if you can use it or see a counselor if that works for you. The events are what they are, and your initial reaction is what it was. The lasting effects, good or bad, will largely depend on how you explain it to yourself. You can't invent a story that ended differently or deny what you felt or did. Your choice is whether you will think, "It should have been me that died; I'm scum." Or "I lived, I was lucky, I did okay; what will I do better if it happens again?"

Stories again. I use stories as a metaphor because I have listened to so many people rewrite their history and edit events and meanings. Not lying, usually the actual events were pretty much as described, but what the events meant and connections between events are artfully altered so that the story, the life made sense.

The world doesn't care if it makes sense or not. The media's "senseless violence" made perfect sense to the person who perpetrated it, yet was possibly a mystery to the victim. The world is big, and chaos is the soul of violence: but humans are the monkeys who must find a pattern. If we can't find one, we will make one. A life story is one metaphor for the pattern we find and create. You could call it a "reality map" just as easily, the picture we hold in our head of how the world works. It is the same—a picture of ourselves or the world often many steps removed from the reality. People will kill and die for their story, usually more easily than they will kill or die for their reality. And damage to the story can be more shattering than damage to their physical bodies.

We are often helped in writing our stories. I talked with an inmate for hours one afternoon. He was a violent sex offender, a drug addict and a veteran of Vietnam. We talked about violence and how it changed the people who lived it and how people who had not experienced violence rarely understood those who had.

When he returned from Vietnam, he was put into counseling with a state psychologist just out of college whose goal was to get him to admit that he had done monstrous things and was a monster. Think about that—for what he was trained, paid, and ordered to do, he was supposed to call himself a monster. It was supposed to help him. The theory came from someone who had no idea of his experiences.

I thought about it for a long time. Violence had had a profound effect on our lives and our personalities. I'm a stable family man. He was a violent addict. How much of that is because he had a state-paid counselor who thought he was a monster and I have a loving wife and a circle of experienced friends? Where would I be if I had been told I was a monster by the people trying to help (and no mistake, I've been called worse, just not by people who mattered to me). Where would he be if the psychologist had just had the wisdom to listen and help him sort it out in his own way?

There are big things and when they happen we expect them to have big effects. Death, life, heroics and cowardice, blood and piss and a grown man's tears or screams. We expect these events to *mean something*, but they don't, not right away. It takes a while, but the transition is when the event becomes a part of you. Not something that happened to you, but a part of you.

The transition can take time and it can look like depression or even obsession. It can become depression or obsession if you let it. Focus on living, stay busy, think about it, but don't try to hold the memory tight, and you will become much stronger.

What is your worst memory? How much impact did that event have on making you into you? Didn't your greatest strengths come from your worst times? Didn't your capacity for compassion arise from your losses and grief? Didn't your courage come from pain?

More specific. One of the most unexpected things about serious violence is that it is not over, ever. Anything that you have done, anything that you have not done, whether it succeeded or failed, will weigh on your mind. In all probability, it will eat at you.

It can be called "survivor's guilt" or "Post-Traumatic Stress Disorder." It can be more debilitating than the incident. The statistics for suicide among survivors and among rescuers is sobering. Many people can't return to the place where the incident happened. The stress on friendships and relationships is immense.

People will look at you strangely. In their mind, they are curious and concerned. They want to ask, "What was it like?" and "Are you okay?" but they are afraid that would be rude, so they say nothing.

You see the look and the silence and interpret it as accusation or fear. Another friend drifts away.

Get counseling. It does help. Talk to a professional. Seek out people who have been through similar things. The law enforcement community has an advantage—they both recognize the phenomenon and have a larger pool of experience with situations that went bad. It is easier for them to find people who have been through this.

It also helps to help others.

I'm going to give you some advice. It is not a substitute for talking to a professional but it will help:

Contact the rest of the survivors the next day. Talk and listen.

Talk to your significant other, your family, and your friends. Don't leave them to imagine what you went through and don't build up a silence of misunderstanding. Not talking is the emotional equivalent of choosing to do nothing during the event.

Whatever you are feeling IS NORMAL! Anyone who tells you differently is full of shit. These situations are so rare that there will never be a standard response. There are some responses that are more common. That is all.

section 7.3: for supervisors

If you are a supervisor, responsible for either the victim group or the rescue/relief team, get some professional help in there. The most common model is the Post-Incident Debriefing. Gather everyone involved and have them talk. It may seem uncomfortable or stilted at first, but it breaks down that first big barrier, the silence. It goes much smoother with an experienced facilitator.

In some instances and with some groups, there may be legal ramifications. It should be kept confidential, but in most cases there is no privileged communication in the debriefing. Make sure that everyone understands that anything said could come up in court. This is especially important if the victims had to resort to lethal force to protect themselves from the threat.

The best facilitator I know, Bill Gatzke, would end the debriefing with a clipboard. He would explain that no one would be in top form for the next little while and ask if there was any business he could take care of: kid's dental appointments, time trades at work, postponing meetings. He got it all taken care of and it was deeply appreciated.

Almost everyone involved will have an urgent need to contact family. Make it happen.

section 7.4: cumulative events

I wrote the following early in 2003. It was purely an attempt to get some stuff out of my head and on to paper where other people could poke at it. The essay included only about half of the stuff that happened that year. There was a case I couldn't talk about, the suicide of a friend, and some other stuff. It took about two years to really settle, and those years were almost as intense as 2002.

BAGGAGE

Experience comes with baggage. Do you really want to know what floats through my head? Here are some images. No particular order, no particular theme.

"Surely we're beyond such quaint notions as 'good' and 'evil,'" she said, and I knew that she had no idea that the blood in a two-year-old baby could cover the walls in every room of a two-story apartment. Sometimes it's hard to know some things.

I've fought someone five inches taller and at least thirty pounds heavier, someone who got the first move at close range...and I was bored. Planning the paperwork while fully engaged.

I just don't react to adrenaline like I used to. Deep in a new cave, fiddling with a knot on my climbing partner's harness, standing on a narrow ledge with my back to a chasm of unknown depth, my finger slipped off the knot with a snap and I started to fall. Both of my partners yelped. I reached out, grabbed one of their shirts and pulled myself back onto balance. No adrenalin—when I went back to the knot my hand wasn't shaking. What's the point of climbing, caving, or kayaking if there's no rush? I might as well be at work.

UFC competitor, Navy Seal, Thai kickboxer, PCP freaks, nutballs with cell-made maces, bikers, killers—all the same effect, no rush. I tell them not to make me hurt them. Most listen. Some don't and they get hurt. But I'd fight any of that list any day rather than another methed-up 300-pound naked woman who had that smell...You know that rotten cheese smell that really obese people with poor hygiene have? Combine it with the smell of rotten fish. No adrenaline, maybe, but I was ready to gag.

The crook was trying to make a show in front of his buddies. "I'm a Golden Gloves boxer," he said, "what are you gonna do?"

I was tired and bored. I told him exactly what I was going to do: "Put you face down in the concrete and make you cry like a little bitch. Now are you going to sit down or am I going to sit you down?" He sat.

I sat down to write a report and my hand was shaking a little. First time in years. No massive, crazed killer—a skinny crack whore with Hepatitis C *and* active tuberculosis tried to bite me. I think I was responding to the bite. Her attempt to gouge my eyes wasn't really that special.

The shooting. Rubber bullets are supposed to hurt a lot and bounce off. The crazy, barricaded crook had made armor for himself, so I fired at one of the two bare patches of skin I could see. I aimed at the thigh first, decided that it might bounce into his groin and I'd be accused of shooting him in the groin deliberately, so I switched the target to his opposite lower leg at the edge of the shin. The whole sequence, opening the door, aiming, changing my mind about the target; aiming again and firing took less than a second. Over the sights, I saw the flesh erupt in a little volcano of blood and meat. It seemed to take up the whole visual field. I racked another round. For days, the thought would roll into my head, "Hey, you shot somebody." A friend of fifteen years said, "I know how you've trained and I know what you do but until you actually shot that guy, I never felt afraid around you. I do now." Another friend drifts away.

It doesn't hurt as bad as the friends who aren't allowed to talk to me—the old climbing buddy whose wife answered the phone one day, "He can't go climbing with you. He's a grown man with responsibilities now and he's not interested in your childish bullshit." The phone slammed down.

I got a call about six in the morning, a friend who has it together, a true professional, and I'm at his house by eight, and he's drunk off his ass and his wife's wedding ring is on the kitchen table. It takes a toll. He does the same job I do; he does it as well as I do, and I am sitting here at his breaking point. Where's my breaking point? Where is my marriage's?

My home life is great and terrifying. My wife has been having incapacitating dizzy spells. MRI, etc. shows nothing. Almost all possible causes have been eliminated except stress, and I'm the only source of stress in her life. I go home to two wonderful children who happen to be autistic. They are "high functioning" but we won't know for years if they will be able to survive on their own in the real world. Did I cause that, too?

I drink too much and don't care. My stomach is always in an uproar and I don't care. After all the fights and decades of training, I finally had my first surgery—ACL. Now my shoulder hurts like hell, not because of anything—it's aggravated by using a mouse and keyboard. What horseshit.

I rarely sleep for more than four hours at a time. Usually, I snap awake for no reason. Sometimes, between CERT, teaching Jujutsu, and Search and Rescue, four hours is all I have. I've been so tired that the muscles in my face were twitching. I could feel it, like ants crawling under the skin, but no one could see it.

It was a great day to be alive. Low, stormy clouds swirled around the cliffs in the gorge and I was alive and the poor son of a bitch in the body bag wasn't. My first body recovery since volunteering for Search and Rescue. It was a good starter body—fresh, not too fat, stiff enough to roll easily but not all splayed out. The inside of his skull was dark and empty. The Medical Examiner had warned me about stepping in the brains. "Slipperiest shit in the world," he said. The corpse had taken (Jumped? Pushed? Accident? I will never know) a hundred-foot face plant onto a sharp basalt boulder. I rappelled the body down to the road. It smelled like fresh meat and Ivory soap. When I got back to my wife's friends, they were resentful that my pager had spoiled their plans to spend the night playing *Uno* or *Trivial Pursuit* or *Balderdash* or something. They spent the next half hour not talking to me. My wife, bless her heart, then decided that playing a new board game called *Zombie* would cheer everybody up. Got to play with dead bodies twice in one day. When I got home, I realized I still had a smear of human goo on my sleeve.

Not just death, life too. When you're holding a newborn baby who is addicted to both crack and heroin and you know it's the mother's seventh...the "miracle of birth" kind of tarnishes.

Martial arts, first Judo and then Jujutsu, have always been my anchor in times like these. When all else was chaos, when I didn't know where to turn, I could always go and sweat and bleed and learn. I don't know where to go now. It is so rare to learn something that works that is new. I'm teaching, but when I look for another instructor for myself, it's as if I'm some kind of alien. Or as if someone who has never seen it is trying to sell me paintings of my own home. Is there an instructor out there who can show me the next step? Is there a next step? Who else has been further down this path? I play; I like playing with people that roll hard. But BJJ or JKD or MMA or FMA is not what I do and not what I need. It's stress relief, an amusing game. For what I do, for what I need, I can't help feeling that I've peaked and don't know where to turn.

You know the lotus-eaters? The ones who believe that what they learn in the *dojo* is exactly like real life? "It's unfair to say that your experience is in some way more valid than my training." Or "the way the people with experience throw it in the face of those of us that don't have it." I sometimes wonder what it would be like arguing from the other side. I like who I am, and the experience has done much to form that...but it would be nice to sleep a full night, and there are some things in my head that aren't very comfortable. Wouldn't it be nice to remember the feel of victory and just forget the screams and smells?

I understand that I'm not changing the world. I don't think, sometimes in my deepest heart of hearts, that I'm even protecting anyone. I think that I'm part of a huge veil; a group of men and women who deal with one tiny aspect of this world so that no one else has to admit it exists. That I exist just so that wealthy, fat, state-educated people can believe that evil is a "quaint notion." I'm holding one finger in the dyke and smiling for the tourists who believe that it is water on the other side.

Most of this was 2002, and I'd hoped for 2003 to be better. At least a bit less intense. In the first two weeks, I waded through a slough looking for the dismembered remains of a teenager, and an officer, someone I know, was shot in the face.

Same old same old.

About the essay. At first reading, it can seem like I was or am clinically depressed. That wasn't what was going on. Birth and death and shootings and divorces are supposed to mean something. These were big things and it took a while for them to change from events into history, from things that happened to me into things that were a part of me. Don't worry about it.

Keep this in perspective: I'm a jail guard who volunteers with Search and Rescue. I'm not a traffic enforcement officer who has had to use a snow shovel to scrape the remains of a pedestrian off the pavement, or a detective who has to develop rapport with rapists again and again, or a paramedic who has seen more shattered bodies in a year than I have or will see in my lifetime. Somewhere, not too far from where you live, there are people who deal with this, people for whom this is part of their everyday world. They do this job so that other people don't have to see it or deal with it or understand it. They carry the baggage of the rhinoceros so that the rest of the world can believe in unicorns.

section 7.5: dealing with the survivor/ student

Sooner or later every martial arts instructor will have a student join for the specific reason of getting over a traumatic assault. Ostensibly, they want the skill and ability to prevent the incident from recurring. More deeply, they want to grow into a person who would not have been a victim.

I get harsh here—if you choose to get involved in this for your ego or reputation, you have absolutely NO BUSINESS teaching or pretending to teach self-defense. If you have no idea what a real attack is like, you can be a danger to students—especially to recent victims who are in a vulnerable state and don't have the experience or objectivity to evaluate your advice. This person has been a victim and is at high risk to be victimized again, and his or her goal is to change that probability. It is not a place for amateurs or pretenders.

People don't break, but everyone, including the survivor/student, is compelled to think that she can be "fixed." She can't. She has reactions based on her experiences and they are completely natural. These reactions, however, are making her life less pleasant than she wants. In order to change the reactions, she has to grow, not mend. She is choosing to do this, so she has to direct the growth.

Counseling is one good and valid option. For a time in college I explored the idea of counseling. My experience with professional counselors at that time was that their therapeutic goal was almost never to change the patient as much as to make the patient comfortable with where they were... resulting in no change, but sometimes an increase in happiness/comfort. The survivors who choose training over counseling or in addition to counseling want change, not accommodation. They want growth.

Growth and change of this magnitude is hard. Why is a caterpillar wrapped in silk while it is changing into a butterfly? So the other caterpillars can't hear the screams. Change hurts.

There are two questions that you must ask the survivor and both of you, survivor and instructor, have to live up to the contract in those words.

"Do you want to get over this?" This is her contract that will be used over and over again to remind her that SHE wanted to change and she was willing to pay the price. There is great power in the victim identity. Instructors and other students go out of their way to be accommodating and gentle. The survivor can often get out of any drill or derail the entire class by admitting her discomfort. This sentence allows the instructor to point it out when this happens, to point out that the benefits of victim status must be given up to outgrow the victim status. This is hard, but critical. The subtle power in the victim status often seems like the only good thing and the only survival tool to come out of the event. Many are reluctant, very reluctant, to give up a useful "victim identity" for a *possible* stronger self.

The second question is: "Do you trust me?" This is critical. Without trust, this can't work. If the trust is betrayed, the damage will be immeasurable. In order for the training to progress, you will have to find the survivor's buttons, the damaged places in her psyche, and push them. You must be ready to say, "That's an excuse, and I'm not going to accept it."

Everything has to be presented as a conscious, intellectual choice between growth and surrender. Intellect is her only way forward. If she goes with her guts and her feelings, she will find a comfortable place and hide there forever. That is a good, valid choice... but she has already said that she doesn't want to keep hiding and running. She can't do both. At every crossroads, she must choose whether to face or run.

Caveat: This does not mean that if she is jogging and gets a bad feeling she should ignore it. Her intuition might have saved her before. It means that she chooses times and places, like martial arts training, to force the screaming little monkey in her head to join the world. She wants her intuition at full speed and full power, but the level of fear she is feeling is not real and actually hampers intuition.

She needs to be constantly reminded that what happened to her is not who she is. That she has friends and a life and millions of other moments in her life that were not that moment. That not one of her friends likes her because of what happened but only because of who she is. And to respect, possibly, that many of her best qualities might have been a result of her worst moments (be careful with that one, but it is an important insight).

Also, if she lets that incident control her life, the rapist is still victimizing her. Which brings up another thought: This incident only has the power that the survivor gives it. In most cases the physical trauma will have healed long before she sought out training. Not everyone has the same reactions to rape. She should, at some point, look at how she sees and remembers the incident, what it means to her, and then very carefully separate her perceptions (attributed meanings) from the reality.

She should (another hard one) look at what benefits she gets from seeing herself as a victim. This is important, because there are very few benefits from being attacked. By identifying oneself as a victim, you can gain great power over compassionate people. Victims have been able to take control not only of their participation in the class but to alter the course of an entire class by expressing discomfort or experiencing flashbacks. This is power for people who have been made to feel powerless and it can be addictive. The student must face the need to give up this power as part of the overall growth.

section 7.6: changes

Exposure, especially repeated exposure to extreme violence, will change you. At the best, the fear of death and the decision to fight will clarify in your mind what is worth fighting for and what is worth dying for. That clarity is very powerful. You will realize how many people are attached to ideas and opinions that are meaningless, and how many of the passionate disagreements of your past were largely pointless.

It may become hard to talk to people. Your frame of reference may have shifted forever. For me, it is hard to care about grown men making millions playing children's games for TV, or the personal lives of people who I will never meet, or political parties that I can't see a substantial difference between.

It's hardest of all to talk to martial artists, to see their shiny happy eyes as they discuss a fantasy that you pray they will never test.

Other things have changed you in the past and will in the future. They are more common things than violence, so they lack the mystique, but they have changed you and will change you just as profoundly. The loss of a childhood pet. Your first love. Becoming a parent. The death of a relative or close friend. Saving a life.

Enlightenment and combat. There are a handful of people who have been faced with a situation, sometimes in combat (but not always), when their death was certain and they fully realized it. In that one instant, if they were lucky enough to survive, they came to fully understand what was important. It was a pure ordering of priorities with absolute certainty that your own life was no longer on the table.

This true acceptance of death changed the person. They could act decisively because they knew what was and what wasn't important. They didn't show or feel fear in quite the same way.

In medieval Japan, the only way to retire from a life as a *bushi* was to enter a monastery. It lead to a large percentage of people, concentrated in temples, who had had this experience—but none of them got it in the temple.

The side effect for martial artists seeking enlightenment (and how do you know you want it anyway? What are the odds that the real world will be more comfortable than your subconscious, self-protective fantasy?) is that they come to believe that they can get to the same place if they mimic the training—but it was the experience, not the training, that brought them there.

My Enlightenment. Lao Tsu said that anyone who talked about *the way* didn't understand it—then he proceeded to write a book on it, so take his advice for what it is worth.

At the library, there are dozens of books on spiritual growth, the Tao, and enlightenment. They all sound the same. They have a shared idea of what is deep and what is profound. The books on tape share a soft-spoken, educated, privileged voice. They talk with reverence of nature. If you meet them, the people who make a living by pointing *the way*, they always have soft hands.

I was raised with many people of deep wisdom. Most not only reverenced nature but had spent much of their life living close to it or wrested their living from the land on ranches or in forests or mines. Their hands were never soft. They rarely spoke. They listened, and you learned to listen in their presence.

I'll tell you of my moment of enlightenment (but be careful, since we have all been told that it can't be explained). While white water rafting at the age of seventeen, I was flipped and trapped under a waterfall. Despite wet suit and flotation vest, I was pressed hard against the riverbed. I was down long enough to not just realize that I was going to die—and there was nothing I could do about it—but for the fact to sink in.

I didn't want to die, but in a second or so I realized that didn't matter, since once I was dead my identity, including my wish to live, would be obliterated. In a matter of a minute or so, it wouldn't matter to me.

I moved on, then, thinking of my poor friends who would miss me, but in ten years I would just be, at most, a painful memory. In twenty or thirty years, no one would remember me. I didn't matter.

In perhaps a hundred years, no one would remember these friends or my family. They, too, would be obliterated. They didn't matter.

In a thousand years or ten thousand, no one would remember my nation. It, too, would share in oblivion and prove to not matter, to never have mattered.

The same for my species, and the earth, the universe, and God. When the last star winks out, none of it will have mattered—and in ten billion years, I will still be nothing—and equal to God.

That was the first stage in my enlightenment: to understand that nothing matters. Hence, everything is equal.

Since I was going to die and it didn't matter, I had the freedom to choose how to die for no other reason than my personal preference: would I prefer to die with calm acceptance or to fight against the inevitable purely for the sake of fighting? I admired fighters, so I fought, and dragged myself across the rocks of the riverbed beyond the undertow, and lived.

This is the part that authors have a hard time with—describing the clarity of perception in the moments after *satori*. You know that you can crush rocks in your hands, run up cliffs. You can hear individual insects under specific rocks on the other side of the valley, colors are clear and so are humans. It is also not important. It's just kind of cool.

To sum up—nothing matters, but some stuff matters to me. Artificial priorities disappear; meaningless questions ("Why are we here?") are outed as time-wasting, self-indulgent, self-centered bullshit. Buddhists speak of attachment. Attachment is the "therefore" (e.g., "I love you, therefore..."). You must love me back? Not likely. Nothing bad must happen to you? Can't control the universe, partner.

So I love because I love without expectation of results or even meaning. I spend time with the people I enjoy having in my world and when they move on, they move on. I act the way I would be proud to act, not to set an example or because I should, but because it pleases me. I like strong people; I will be strong. I like skillful people; I will develop skill. I like people who take care of others; I will protect and defend and if I die doing the job, cool—because I am going to die anyway and nothing will ever have mattered.

I can't give promises or guarantees. I can't give comfort with a clean conscience. What I give my students are percentage points, an edge. The most realistic picture I can of what they might face and the strategies that have worked for me over time. I talk from the first day about luck and chaos, and the psychological and emotional blocks to their own actions. I tell them what they might go through during and after an assault in hopes that the prepared mind will heal faster.

BIBLIOGRAPHY

First off, read a damn book. Read lots of books. When you commute, listen to recorded books and when you have dead time and no real life around you to watch, crack open a book. Read as much as you can on as many subjects as you can and keep both a skeptical and an open mind. Let the new ideas in, play with them, but don't just swallow them whole. Just because it got published doesn't mean it's true.

Read more non-fiction than fiction. The world is a huge and amazing place and in history and anthropology you will find weirdness and drama that puts fiction to shame. And you will gain some insight, because everything connects.

Many of the books you read will have bibliographies. Bibliographies will lead you to more information. Often the sources quoted go into much more detail on a single aspect of the issue than was presented in the book.

What follows is a list of books that I got some things out of. It won't be complete. I try to read two non-fiction books a week and in the course of the last few decades I must have forgotten hundreds of titles.

Furthermore, there isn't an author on this list that I agree with 100%. Be skeptical. Check sources. Sometimes you will find that the sources quoted do not say what the author says. That's life in the big city.

I have a website at chirontraining.com, I do most of my thinking out loud at chirontraining.blogspot.com

About people:
Morris, Desmond. *Manwatching*. Harry N Abrams, 1979.
Morris, Desmond. *The Naked Ape*. Delta, 1999.

> Desmond Morris applies his skill as a primatologist to understanding humans and it works uncomfortably well. This is a critical book for looking at people, including yourself, with a fresh eye. In a similar way, Marvin Harris' *Cows, Pigs, Wars and Witches* looks at cultural institutions.

Bernstein, Albert J. *Emotional Vampires*. McGraw-Hill 2002.

> This is an introduction to personality disorders. The book deals with the low-level disorders that make other people's lives miserable. But increase the intensity a bit and you get many of the flavors of criminal behavior.

Siebert, Al. *The Survivor Personality*. Perigee Trade, 1996.

> Not sure you could use this book to develop the traits of a survivor, but if you already have the personality it's a big help in explaining why you don't always connect with other people. That's what I got out of it.

Keirsey and Bates. *Please Understand Me*. Prometheus Nemesis Book Company, 1984.

> Again, different ways of looking at the world mean different ways of being human. The ability to recognize, understand and adapt your communication style to another personality type is key to avoiding conflict.

About Criminals:

Samenow, Stanford. *Inside the Criminal Mind*. Crown, 2004.

> Samenow gets some flack because his views seem harsh, but this is the best description I've read in a long time about how criminals think.

Allen, Bud and Bosta Diana. *Games Criminals Play*. Rae John Publishers, 1981.

> If you spend time with criminals, this is a must read. It shows, in detail, how long-term manipulation happens; how criminals see you and how they try to use you.

Rhodes, Richard. *Why They Kill*. Vintage, 2000.

> An introduction to the works of criminologist Lonnie Athens. His "violentization" process covers the facts I know about people becoming criminals better than anything I've read. His insights on working off the blue print and the mental community have influenced the way I see the world greatly.

Fleisher, Mark S. *Beggars and Thieves*. University of Wisconsin Press, 1995.

> The best book I've read on the low-level hustlers and habitual criminals. Fleisher put words to things that were right in front of my face for years.

About Training:

Beck, Tobi. *The Armored Rose*. Beckenhall Publications, 1999.

It's supposed to be sport-specific to heavy armored combat in the Society for Creative Anachronism, but Ms. Beck's insights on female psychology have really helped me as a trainer and I've used her information on differences in adrenalization between genders to plan tactical operations.

Siddle, Bruce. *Sharpening the Warrior's Edge*. PPCT Research Publications, 1995.

This book is a compilation and interpretation of available research on the survival stress response (SSR), the adrenaline dump that accompanies sudden assault.

About Crime:

Davis, Debra Anne. Betrayed by the Angel. *Harvard Review* Nov./Dec, 2004.

This is a short article available on the web. Ms. Davis poignantly and frankly describes her rape. It was critical to my understanding that all the skill in the world will not help unless you give yourself permission to use it.

Strong, Sanford. *Strong on Defense*. Atria, 1997.

Lt. Strong does an excellent job of describing some of the worst crimes and explaining strategies that have been successful for survivors.

Aftermath:

Artwohl and Christensen. *Deadly Force Encounters*. Paladin Press, 1997.

When CERT was making the transition from an unarmed/Less-lethal team to a fully armed hostage rescue team, this book was required reading. The authors, now a retired police psychologist and a retired officer, were uniquely placed to get good information on what officers in deadly force encounters had experienced and thought before, during and after the event.

Loren Christensen is a retired cop, a champion *karateka* and a prolific author. His works cover everything from gangs and prostitution to defensive tactics, to combat ethics and how to train. With his unique combination of training and experience, any of his books are worth a look: www.lwcbooks.com

Shay, Jonathan. *Achilles in Vietnam*. Simon & Schuster, 1995.

Shay describes pretty extreme cases of PTSD, but points out that this is not new and points out where the damage comes and some of how it can be prevented.

Kirschman, Ellen. *I Love a Cop*. Guilford Press, 2006.

This is a book written for police families to prepare them for the changes that their loved one will go through. As such it is a powerful book about the effect of long term exposure to a violent world.

Kirkham, George. *Signal Zero*. Lippincott, 1976.

A professor who used to teach the 70's mantra that a certain sub-human personality type was drawn to the law enforcement career is challenged by a student to be a street cop for a time. A powerful book by someone who has lived and seen the prejudices that the denizens of the violent and the peaceful worlds have about each other.

Other:

DeBecker, Gavin. *The Gift of Fear*. Little, Brown and Company, 1997.

A book about intuition. Very valuable.

Gonzales, Laurence. *Deep Survival*. W. W. Norton and Company, 2004.

This book is about why some people die. How fixation on a plan can get you killed, when habitual competence can get you killed—there were a number of good insights in here and even a few 'wake-up calls'.

Marc "Animal" MacYoung. *The Professional's Guide to Ending Violence Quickly*. Paladin Press, 1996.

This was required reading for CERT while we were a primarily hand-to-hand team. I like the way Marc thinks about violence and his descriptions of experiences and how they affected him match my own more than any other author. All of his books are worth a read. He maintains a Web site at www.nononsenseselfdefense.com. The site seems very rambling. If there is one thing you have learned from this book, it is that violence is complicated. His Web site seems to respect that fact.

Grossman, Lt. Col. Dave. *On Killing.* Back Bay Books, 2003.

Grossman, Lt. Col. Dave and Loren Christensen. *On Combat.* PPCT Research Publications, 2004.

On Killing was a pioneering first step in applying good academic research methodology to the study of human violence. It is a must read. Generally, *On Combat* continued with the theme but was far less accurate in its presentation of sources and more focused on an agenda than getting the information out there. Don't take my word for this. Read the book, then read the sources in the bibliography.

The Bureau of Justice Statistics: http://www.ojp.usdoj.gov/bjs/

This is *the* source for statistical data on crime. If someone presents crime data that seems fishy, check it out here.

Night by Elie Wiesel

Read this book. Read it because it is great literature, but also for three things—to see what the cost can be for ignoring signs and not acting; for seeing what humans are capable of when they are hungry, scared, and hopeless; and to see that great things, great art and great insight can arise from the darkest of human experience.

Ultimate Survivors (video) (Calibre Press 1991).

The story of the murder of Linda Lawrence is a "worst case scenario" of a close quarters battle with a threat in excited delirium. A powerful wake-up call for people who are tempted to extrapolate normal experiences to abnormal situations.

The Murder of Georgia Deputy Kyle Dinkheller (video).   http://www.lineofduty.com

Lineofduty gave me permission to show a piece of this video in my seminars. It is powerful and one of the few things that can consistently make a too-confident young martial artist face the fact that knowing what to do and doing it are two very different things.

Criminals by Criminals:

A number of violent criminals have written books and they are well worth a read, but be very, very careful. One of the hardest things for civilians and even researchers to grasp is that whereas normal people need a reason to lie, criminals need a reason to tell the truth. In a violent, marginal world information is power and disinformation is habit.

So read the books, but keeping mind what the authors have done. The writings are not largely valuable for the descriptions of crimes or how people become criminals or even how they see their victims. The books, almost universally, are about how a criminal will manipulate YOU the reader into believing that he is an ordinary guy or a victim himself or even a hero. Practicing to see this is invaluable.

Books on Self-Defense:

I wanted to leave this section out, but you expect it, so here it is. There is a lot of bad information out there. There is even more good (but limited) information, people who have seen or dealt with a piece of the matrix and are willing to sell you an answer.

I like Loren W. Christensen's books. Loren has been there done that on a level that most people will never achieve. http://www.lwcbooks.com/

Lawrence Kane's *Surviving Armed Assault: A Martial Artists Guide to Weapons, Street Violence and Countervailing Force* (YMAA Publication Center, 2006) is an outstanding introduction to an armed world. He doesn't pretend to supply a lot of answers and I respect that a lot.

Massad Ayoob's *The Truth About Self Protection* (Police Bookshelf, 1983) is a classic. Maybe a bit dated, but accurate.

Are there more? Dozens. Some are good and some might get you killed. I can't recommend a lot of books filled with technique. Hopefully, one thing you have learned from this book is that technique is not the answer. There is no recipe for survival. The answer is almost always inherent in the problem if you can see it and if you act.

Kris Wilder and Lawrence Kane are coming out with a book with the intriguing working title, *The Little Black Book of Violence*. It should be interesting.

Martial Arts:

I've read hundreds of books on this subject over the years. There is a lot to learn—history, culture, technique, strategies- enough to keep you going for a very long time. The most important thing is to get out of it what is there. I read Draeger for history and insight; Bluming for thug philosophy. Yang, Jwing-Ming for Chinese perspectives on the things I see in real life (for everything that happens there are many ways to see and explain it.) I collect old books on Judo and Jujutsu because some of the authors were brutal and knew the line between practice and breaking people. Fairbairn and Applegate for books by two men who taught people how to survive in the bloodiest war of modern history. Books on the history of boxing give insight on how the gloves changed the sport and how safety concerns change strategy.

It gets complex. When you find a nugget of good information, keep it. Here is one piece of advice on reading books on martial arts: read books by arrogant people who unabashedly claim that their art is the best. It won't be complete and it won't necessarily be right, but they will work to show you the best of what their art has to offer.

The Way of Kata: Comprehensive Guide for Deciphering Martial Application by Lawrence Kane and Kris Wilder (YMAA Publication Center, 2005) I do have to make one recommendation especially for anyone who studies an art based on solo kata. Lawrence and Kris do not only a superb job of teaching how to "read" kata, but also tie it in to strategy and remembering what it is all about.

INDEX

ABOUT THE AUTHOR

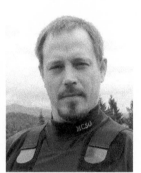

MWM, H/W proportionate, athletic. Non-smoker. ISO insight, new knowledge and, (dare I say?) wisdom. Already found true love. An incurable romantic who believes in doing the right thing, I enjoy long swordfights on the beach, spectacular sunsets in my opponent's eyes, and the feeling of a job well done.

"Sarge is what happens when you raise a kid without a television." —Deputy Rick Hathaway, explaining me to a rookie.

"It's easy to understand Rory if you work from the assumption that he was raised by coyotes." —My wife, who would know better than anybody.

Most everything you want to know about me is in the preface under "The Truth About Me."

From a recent seminar flyer:

"Rory Miller has been studying martial arts since 1981. Though he started in competitive martial sports, earning college varsities in judo and fencing, he found his martial "home" in the early Tokugawa-era battlefield system of Sosuishi-ryu kumi uchi (Jujutsu). He is a veteran corrections officer and with hundreds of unarmed encounters has thoroughly examined the gulf that exists between training and application. In addition to Jujutsu and self-defense, Sgt. Miller teaches and designs courses in Use of Force policy and decision making, Police Defensive Tactics, Confrontational Simulations, Crisis Communication With the Mentally Ill, and leads and trains his agency's Corrections Tactical Team. He has written a few articles for national magazines and he is featured in Loren Christensen's *Fighter's Fact Book 2: The Street.*"

Things I've done most of you haven't:
- Got zapped with a Taser (sucked)
- Zapped somebody with a Taser (probably saved his life)
- Drank chichu with a former cannibal (tasted like watery milky beer)
- Vision quested
- Talked someone down (actually a few) in excited delirium
- Failed to talk even more down in excited delirium
- Taken a knife away from someone who tried to stick it in my back (luck)
- Played patty-cake with a rattlesnake (stupid, but it was a baby)

However, I have never learned to ride a motorcycle or water ski. There's still lots of cool stuff to do.

BOOKS FROM YMAA

6 HEALING MOVEMENTS
101 REFLECTIONS ON TAI CHI CHUAN
A WOMAN'S QIGONG GUIDE
ADVANCING IN TAE KWON DO
ANCIENT CHINESE WEAPONS
ANALYSIS OF SHAOLIN CHIN NA 2ND ED.
ARTHRITIS RELIEF: CHINESE QIGONG FOR HEALING & PREVENTION, 3RD ED.
BACK PAIN RELIEF: CHINESE QIGONG FOR HEALING & PREVENTION 2ND ED
BAGUAZHANG
CARDIO KICKBOXING ELITE
CHIN NA IN GROUND FIGHTING
CHINESE FAST WRESTLING: THE ART OF SAN SHOU KUAI JIAO
CHINESE FITNESS: A MIND / BODY APPROACH
CHINESE TUI NA MASSAGE
COMPLETE CARDIOKICKBOXING
COMPREHENSIVE APPLICATIONS OF SHAOLIN CHIN NA
CONFLICT COMMUNICATION
DUKKHA: A SAM REEVES MARTIAL ARTS THRILLER
DUKKHA REVERB: A SAM REEVES MARTIAL ARTS THRILLER
DUKKHA UNLOADED: A SAM REEVES MARTIAL ARTS THRILLER
EIGHT SIMPLE QIGONG EXERCISES FOR HEALTH, 2ND ED.
ENZAN: THE FAR MOUNTAIN
ESSENCE OF SHAOLIN WHITE CRANE
ESSENCE OF TAIJI QIGONG, 2ND ED.
FACING VIOLENCE
FIGHTING ARTS
INSIDE TAI CHI
KATA AND THE TRANSMISSION OF KNOWLEDGE
LITTLE BLACK BOOK OF VIOLENCE
LIUHEBAFA FIVE CHARACTER SECRETS
MARTIAL ARTS ATHLETE
MARTIAL ARTS INSTRUCTION
MARTIAL WAY AND ITS VIRTUES
MEDITATIONS ON VIOLENCE
MIND/BODY FITNESS: A MIND / BODY APPROACH
THE MIND INSIDE TAI CHI
MUGAI RYU: THE CLASSICAL SAMURAI ART OF DRAWING THE SWORD
NATURAL HEALING WITH QIGONG: THERAPEUTIC QIGONG
NORTHERN SHAOLIN SWORD, 2ND ED.
OKINAWA'S COMPLETE KARATE SYSTEM: ISSHIN RYU
PRINCIPLES OF TRADITIONAL CHINESE MEDICINE

QIGONG FOR HEALTH & MARTIAL ARTS 2ND ED.
QIGONG FOR LIVING
QIGONG FOR TREATING COMMON AILMENTS
QIGONG MASSAGE —FUNDAMENTAL TECHNIQUES FOR HEALTH AND
    RELAXATION, 2ND ED.
QIGONG MEDITATION: EMBRYONIC BREATHING
QIGONG MEDITATION—SMALL CIRCULATION
QIGONG, THE SECRET OF YOUTH
QUIET TEACHER
ROOT OF CHINESE QIGONG, 2ND ED.
SHIN GI TAI—KARATE TRAINING FOR BODY, MIND, AND SPIRIT
SHIHAN TE: THE BUNKAI OF KATA
SIMPLIFIED TAI CHI CHUAN 24 & 48 POSTURES
SUNRISE TAI CHI
SURVIVING ARMED ASSAULTS
TAE KWON DO: THE KOREAN MARTIAL ART
TAEKWONDO BLACK BELT POOMSAE
TAEKWONDO: A PATH TO EXCELLENCE
TAEKWONDO: ANCIENT WISDOM FOR THE MODERN WARRIOR
TAEKWONDO: DEFENSES AGAINST WEAPONS
TAEKWONDO: SPIRIT AND PRACTICE
TAI CHI BALL QIGONG: FOR HEALTH AND MARTIAL ARTS
TAI CHI BOOK
TAI CHI CHIN NA: THE SEIZING ART OF TAI CHI CHUAN
TAI CHI CHUAN CLASSICAL YANG STYLE (REVISED
    EDITION)
TAI CHI CHUAN MARTIAL APPLICATIONS
TAI CHI CHUAN MARTIAL POWER
TAI CHI CONNECTIONS
TAI CHI DYNAMICS
TAI CHI QIGONG, 3RD ED.
TAI CHI SECRETS OF THE ANCIENT MASTERS
TAI CHI SECRETS OF THE WU & LI STYLES
TAI CHI SECRETS OF THE WU STYLE
TAI CHI SECRETS OF THE YANG STYLE
TAI CHI SWORD: CLASSICAL YANG STYLE
TAIJIQUAN THEORY OF DR. YANG, JWING-MING
TENGU: THE MOUNTAIN GOBLIN, A CONNOR BURKE
    MARTIAL ARTS THRILLER
TRADITIONAL CHINESE HEALTH SECRETS
TRADITIONAL TAEKWONDO
WESTERN HERBS FOR MARTIAL ARTISTS
XINGYIQUAN, 2ND ED.

DVDS FROM YMAA

ANALYSIS OF SHAOLIN CHIN NA
ADVANCED PRACTICAL CHIN NA IN DEPTH
BAGUAZHANG 1,2, & 3 —EMEI BAGUAZHANG
CHEN STYLE TAIJIQUAN
CHIN NA IN DEPTH COURSES 1: 4
CHIN NA IN DEPTH COURSES 5: 8
CHIN NA IN DEPTH COURSES 9: 12
EIGHT SIMPLE QIGONG EXERCISES FOR HEALTH
THE ESSENCE OF TAIJI QIGONG
FIVE ANIMAL SPORTS
INFIGHTING
KNIFE DEFENSE—TRADITIONAL TECHINIQUES AGAINST DAGGER
MERIDIAN QIGONG
NEIGONG FOR MARTIAL ARTS
QIGONG FOR HEALING
QIGONG MASSAGE—FUNDAMENTAL TECHNIQUES FOR HEALTH AND
    RELAXATION
SHAOLIN KUNG FU FUNDAMENTAL TRAINING 1&2
SHAOLIN LONG FIST KUNG FU: BASIC SEQUENCES
SHAOLIN SABER: BASIC SEQUENCES
SHAOLIN STAFF: BASIC SEQUENCES
SHAOLIN WHITE CRANE GONG FU BASIC TRAINING 1&2
SIMPLE QIGONG EXERCISES FOR ARTHRITIS RELIEF
SIMPLE QIGONG EXERCISES FOR BACK PAIN RELIEF

SIMPLIFIED TAI CHI CHUAN
SUNRISE TAI CHI
SUNSET TAI CHI
SWORD—FUNDAMENTAL TRAINING
TAI CHI ENERGY PATTERNS
TAIJI BALL QIGONG COURSES 1&2—16 CIRCLING AND 16 ROTATING
    PATTERNS
TAIJI BALL QIGONG COURSES 3&4—16 PATTERNS OF WRAP-COILING &
    APPLICATIONS
TAIJI MARTIAL APPLICATIONS: 37 POSTURES
TAIJI PUSHING HANDS 1&2—YANG STYLE SINGLE AND DOUBLE PUSHING
    HANDS
TAIJI PUSHING HANDS 3&4—MOVING SINGLE AND DOUBLE PUSHING HANDS
TAIJI SABER: THE COMPLETE FORM, QIGONG & APPLICATIONS
TAIJI & SHAOLIN STAFF - FUNDAMENTAL TRAINING
TAIJI YIN YANG STICKING HANDS
TAIJIQUAN CLASSICAL YANG STYLE
TAIJI SWORD, CLASSICAL YANG STYLE
UNDERSTANDING QIGONG 1: WHAT IS QI? • HUMAN QI CIRCULATORY SYSTEM
UNDERSTANDING QIGONG 2: KEY POINTS • QIGONG BREATHING
UNDERSTANDING QIGONG 3: EMBRYONIC BREATHING
UNDERSTANDING QIGONG 4: FOUR SEASONS QIGONG
UNDERSTANDING QIGONG 5: SMALL CIRCULATION
UNDERSTANDING QIGONG 6: MARTIAL QIGONG BREATHING
WHITE CRANE HARD & SOFT QIGONG
YANG TAI CHI FOR BEGINNERS

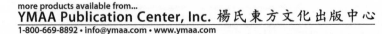

more products available from...
YMAA Publication Center, Inc. 楊氏東方文化出版中心
1-800-669-8892 • info@ymaa.com • www.ymaa.com

Printed in the USA
CPSIA information can be obtained
at www.ICGtesting.com
JSHW022335140824
68134JS00019B/1494